# Deafness

*Designed and produced by*
Aladdin Books Ltd
70 Old Compton Street
London W1V 5PA

*First published in the United States in 1989 by*
Franklin Watts
387 Park Avenue South
New York NY 10016

*Design*: David West Children's Book Design
*Editor*: Zuza Vrbova
*Picture Research*: Cecilia Weston-Baker
*Illustrator*: Stuart Brendon

*Consultant*: Colin Redman on behalf of The National Deaf Children's Society, Great Britain.



Printed in Belgium

Library of Congress Cataloging-in-Publication Data

Taylor, Barbara, 1938-
Living with deafness/by Barbara Taylor.
p. cm.
Includes index.
Summary: Discusses various forms and degrees of deafness, how it may be caused and how it can be treated, and how individuals cope with it.
ISBN 0-531-10842-2
1. Deafness. 2. Hearing. [1. Deaf. 2. Physically handicapped.]
I. Title. II. Title: Deafness.
RF290.T39 1989
617.8--dc20 89-8895
CIP
AC

## CONTENTS

Living with

# Deafness

Barbara Taylor



FRANKLIN WATTS
New York : London : Toronto : Sydney

# HOW THE EAR WORKS

The ear collects vibrations from the air (sounds) and changes them into nerve impulses, which the brain "hears." The outer ear is made up of the pinna and the ear canal. Near its entrance, the ear canal is lined with hairs and wax, which help to keep it clean.

The ear canal leads to a flexible, circular membrane, called the eardrum. When sound waves hit the eardrum, it vibrates. This makes three tiny bones in the middle ear vibrate. These bones make the vibrations stronger and more intensified and pass them on to the inner ear.

The inner ear consists of a complex system of tubes filled with a watery liquid. Vibrations from the middle ear make the liquid move, and sensitive nerve endings convert this movement into electrical signals. These signals are sent to the brain along the nerve of hearing (auditory nerve).

The way in which the electrical signals are interpreted by the brain is not yet clearly understood.

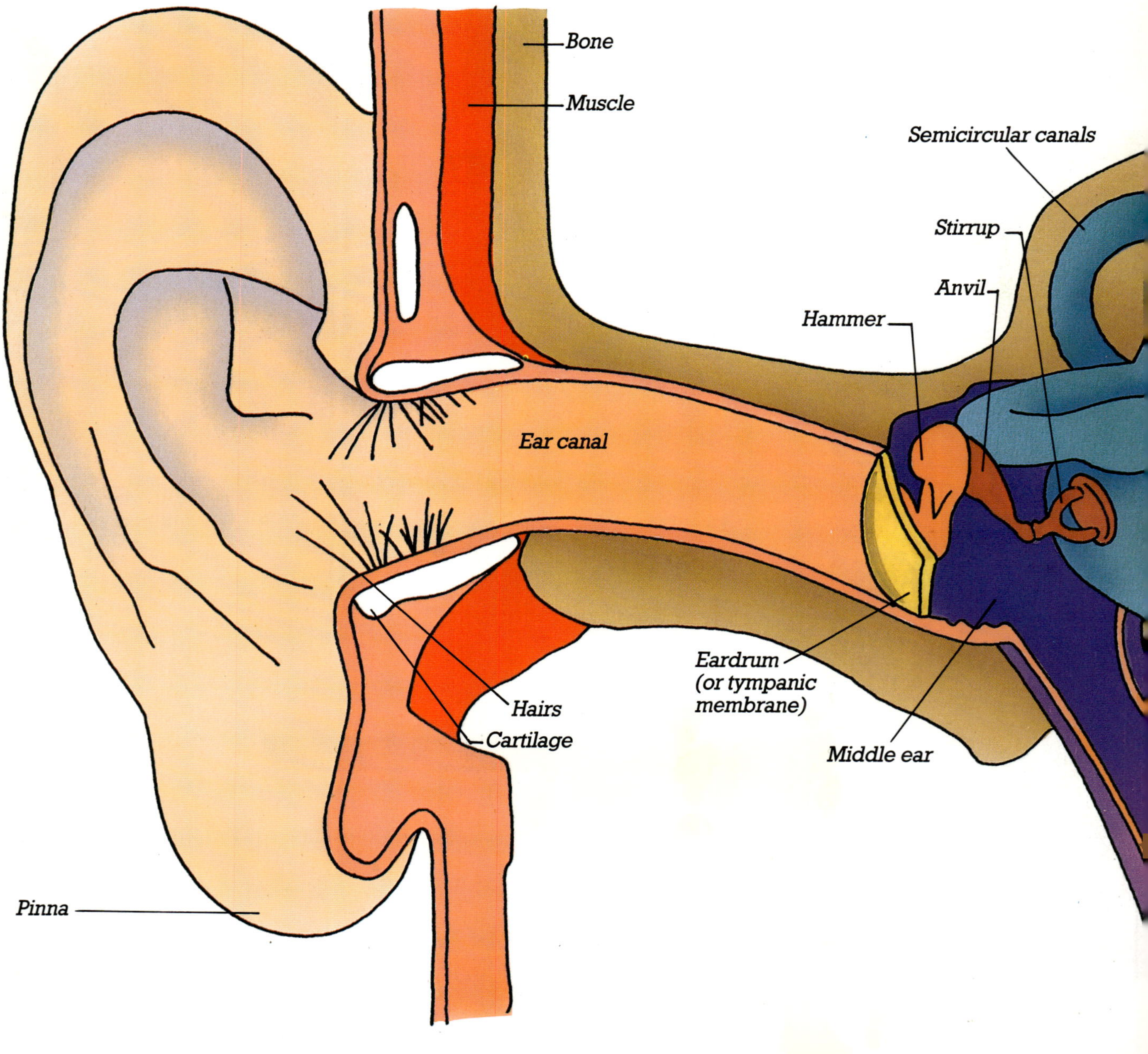

## Seeing sound

Sounds are made when something makes the air shake backwards and forwards very fast. These shaking movements are called vibrations. When air molecules vibrate, they bump against one another. This causes the vibrations to spread through the air in waves – called sound.

Sound waves are invisible but you can see evidence of them if you hold a vibrating tuning fork in some water. The sound waves make the water shake and splash (below).

## Feeling sound

The sounds we make come from the throat. Put one hand against the front of your throat and make a humming noise. Can you feel your throat vibrating? In the same way you can feel the sound of a drum skin vibrating (below). Inside the throat are folds of muscle called vocal cords. When we want to speak or sing, we push air from the lungs past the vocal cords. This makes the cords vibrate and produce sounds. The sounds are shaped into words by your mouth and tongue.

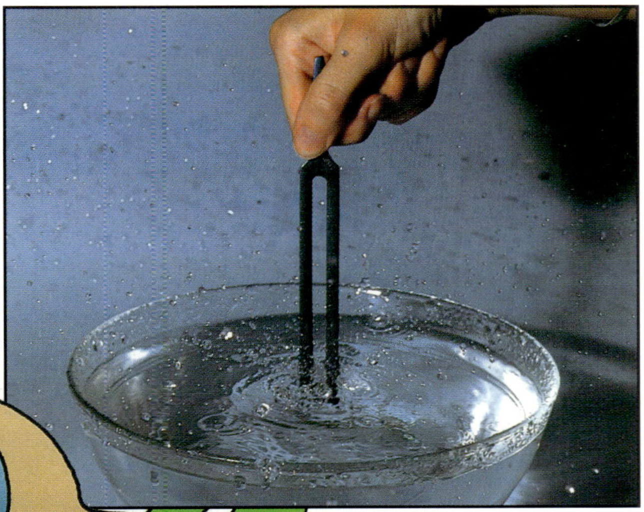

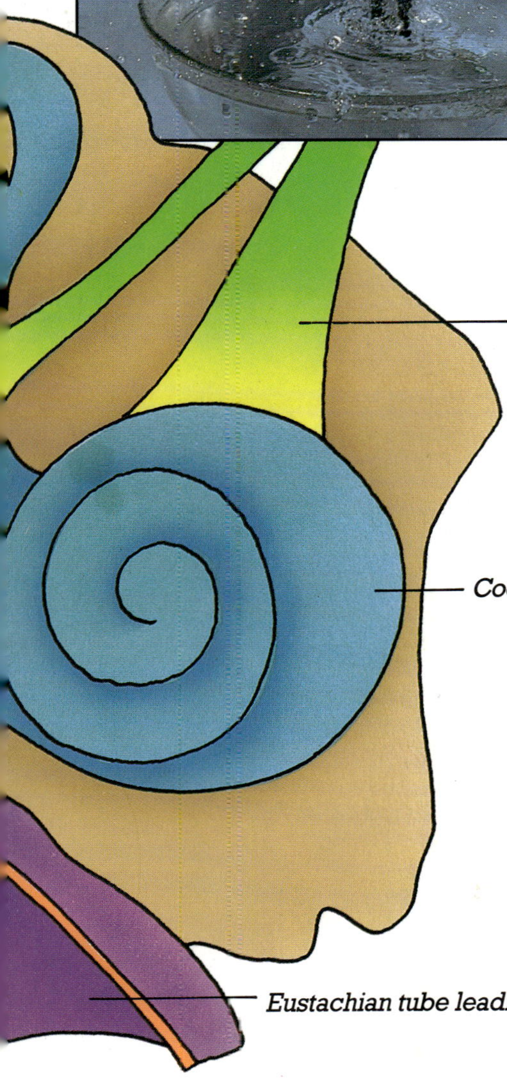


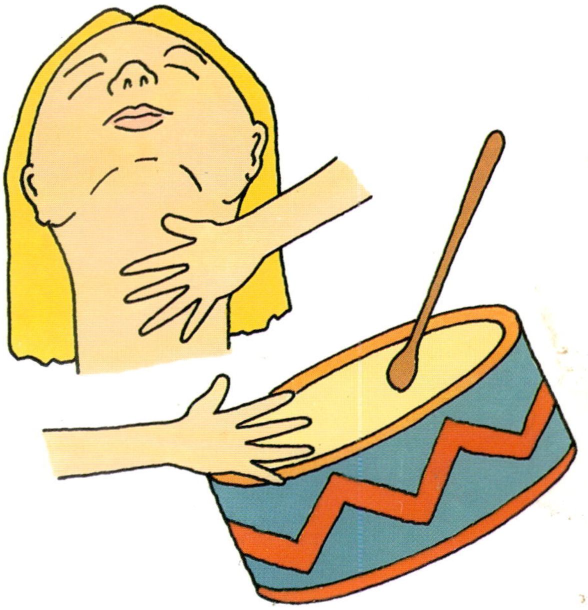

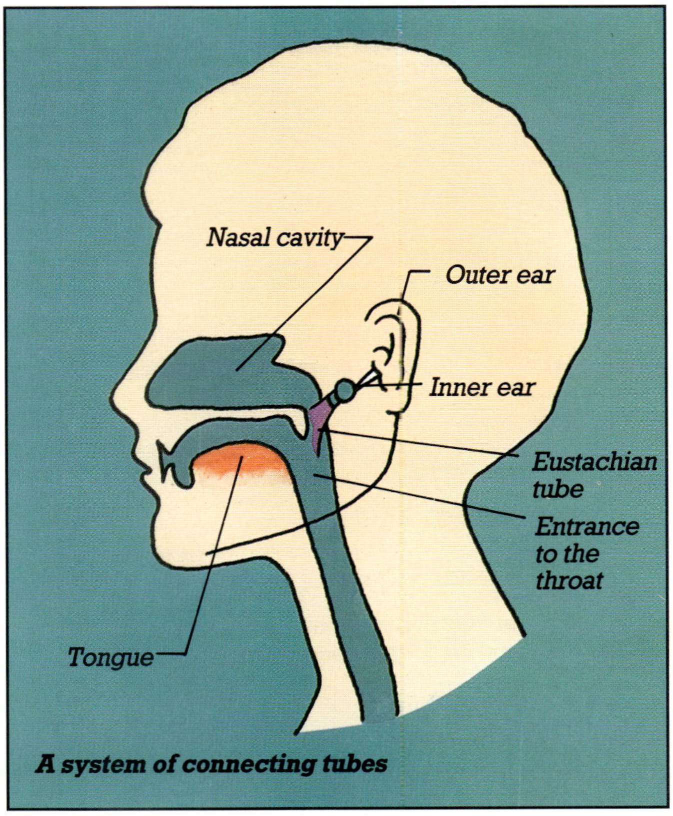


***A system of connecting tubes***

## The smallest bones

The three bones in the middle ear are the smallest bones in the body. Because of their shape, they are called the hammer, anvil and stirrup. They are linked so that the vibrations of one bone can easily make the next bone in the chain vibrate and so send signals to the brain.

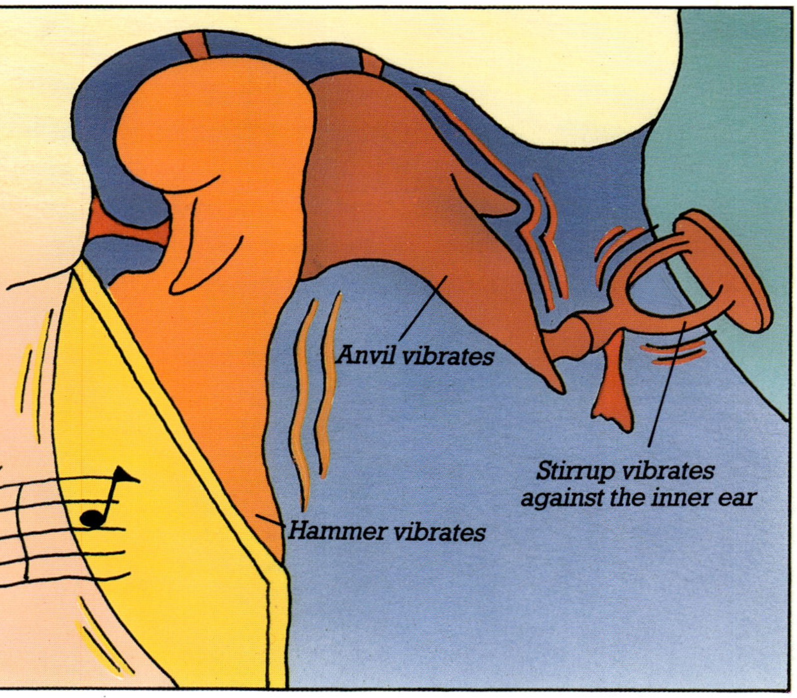


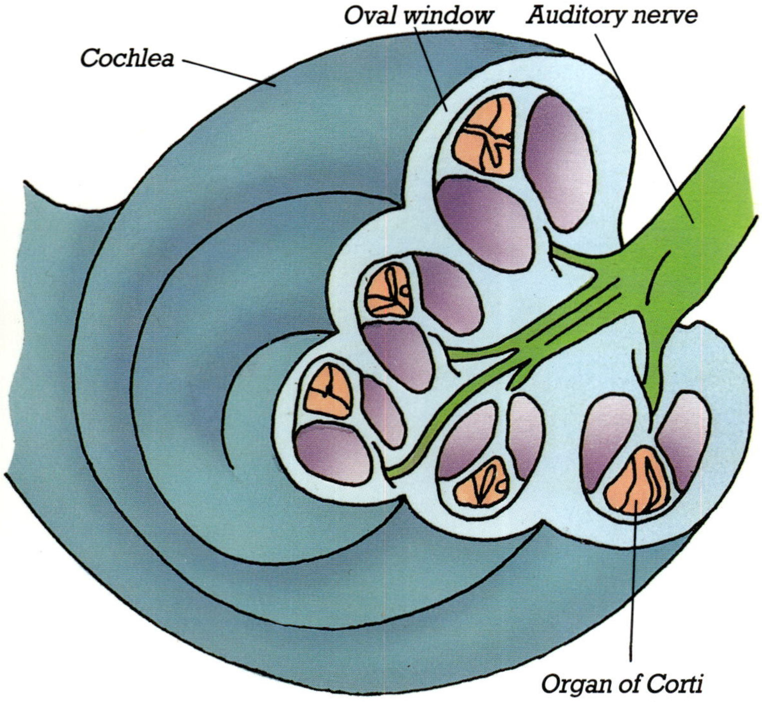


## Sound waves into signals

In the spiral cochlea of the inner ear, the vibrations caused by sound waves in the air are converted into electrical signals. Vibrations enter the cochlea through a membrane called the oval window. They pass into a fluid-filled tube. Altogether it is about as long as your little finger and it is shaped like a snail's shell. The tube contains membranes with thousands of tiny, hair like nerve endings. This is called the Organ of Corti. The vibrations make the fluid move, which bends the hairs and causes the nerves to fire off electrical signals. These signals are sent to the brain along the auditory nerve. Bigger vibrations create louder sounds.

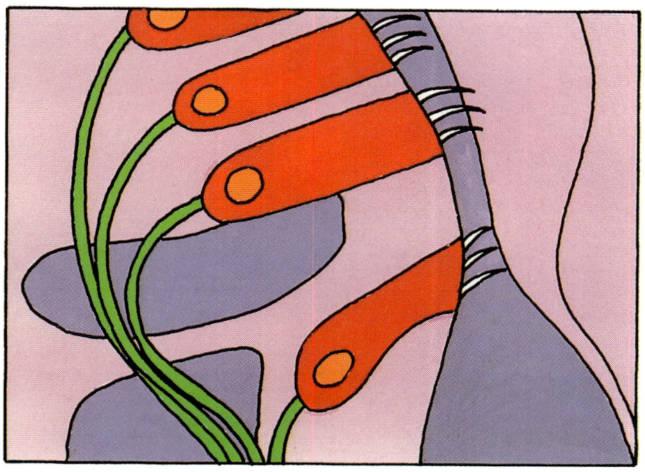

*Sensory hair cells in the Organ of Corti*

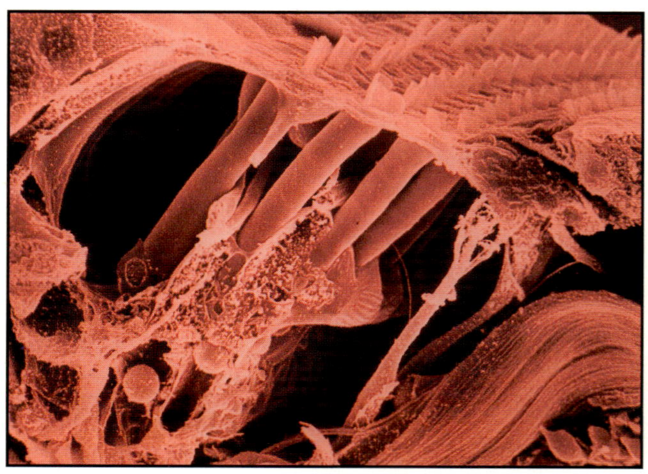

*Electron micrograph of the Organ of Corti*

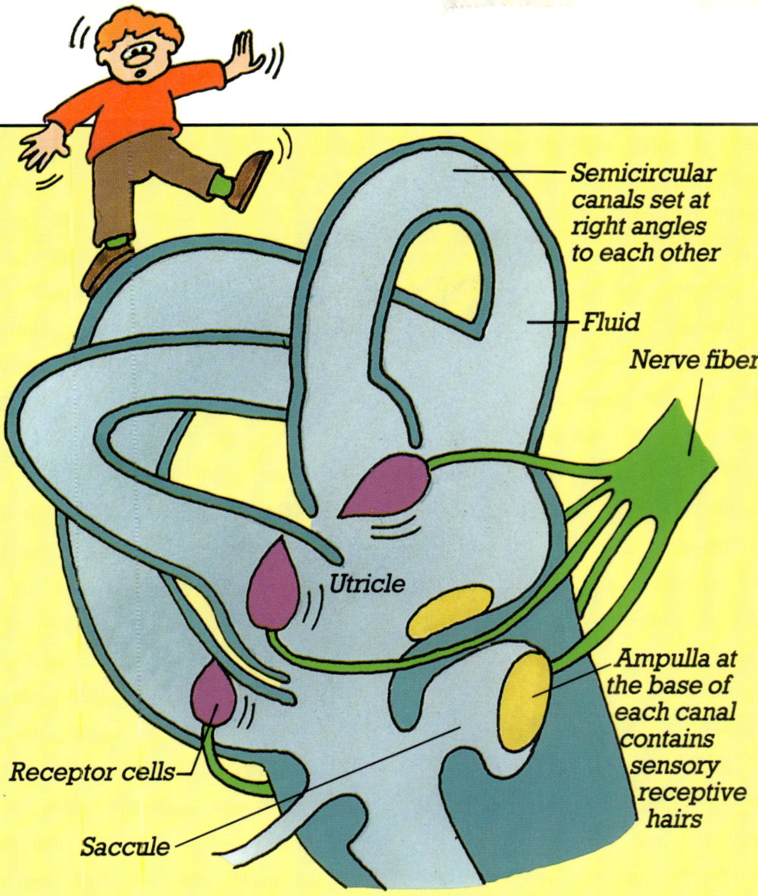


## BALANCE

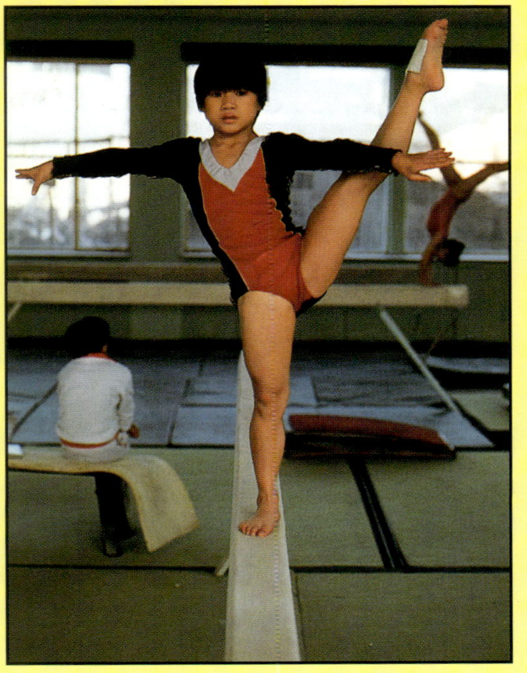

It is the three semicircular canals, in the inner ear, that give you your sense of balance. At one end of each is a swollen area called the ampulla. The semicircular canals open into two sacs called the utricle and the saccule. The whole structure is filled with fluid. The ampulla, utricle and saccule all contain sensory hairs. As you tilt your head, the fluid presses on the hairs, which convert the pressure into electrical signals that travel to the brain. The sacs tell you the position of your head and the canals tell you the direction it is moving. In the utricle and saccule, the tiny hairs are surrounded by a jelly like substance containing minute crystals of calcium carbonate, called otoliths. As the crystals move, under the influence of gravity, they stimulate the hairs, which trigger nerve impulses to the brain.

## HEARING AND THE BRAIN

Signals from the cochlea in the inner ear travel to the brain along the auditory nerve. The nerve carries the sound signals to the base of the brain. This area is called the auditory cortex. Here the brain interprets the signals into "sounds." The way in which sound waves picked up by our ears are actually turned into electrical energy, and interpreted by the brain, is not fully understood.

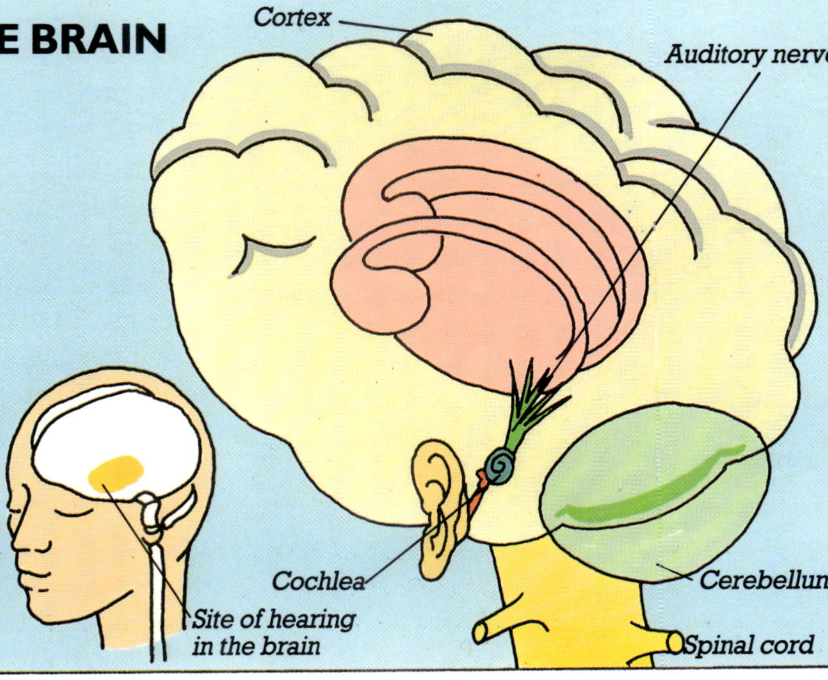

# KINDS OF HEARING PROBLEMS

At least one child in every thousand is born profoundly deaf. Many more people develop hearing impediments later in life because of accidents or diseases.

There are two main kinds of hearing problem. One kind affects the outer or middle ear. This can produce a "conductive" hearing difficulty and it can usually be treated and cured. The other main type of problem that affects people's sense of hearing is connected to the inner ear or the nerve of hearing (auditory nerve). It is called "nerve deafness." Unfortunately, this kind of deafness is usually permanent.

Conductive deafness leads to a loss of loudness, which is like trying to listen to someone who is speaking very quietly or is very far away. Nerve deafness cuts down the loudness and distorts sounds as well. So it is rather like listening to someone speaking an unknown foreign language. This disordered interpretation of sound is a typical symptom of inner ear diseases.

## Blocked ears

One of the simplest causes of hearing loss is the ear canal becoming blocked. This stops some sound waves from reaching the eardrum. Natural wax moves out of the ear all the time to help carry dirt out of the ear. But if this wax becomes hard, it stays in the canal and forms a blockage. A small object which has been pushed into the ear can also block out sound. Because the ear canal is lined with skin, it can also be blocked by skin conditions such as eczema or boils.

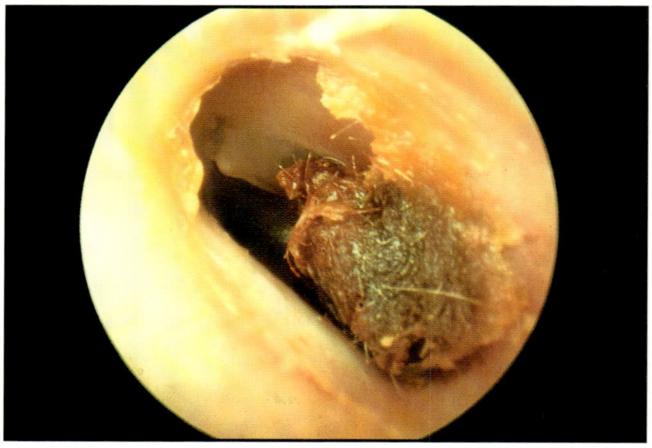

*Ear wax blocking the ear canal*

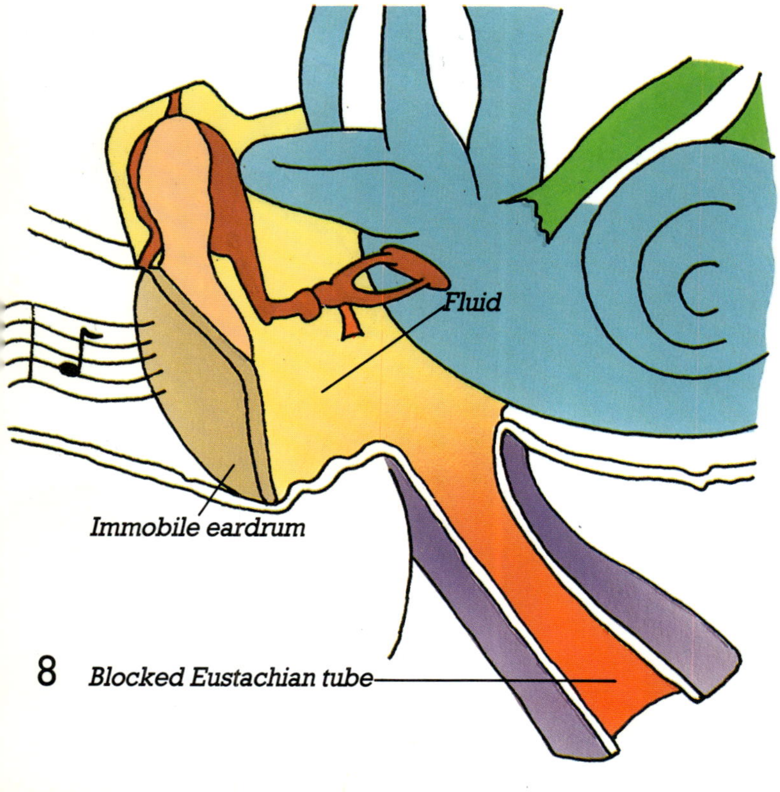


## Glue ear

Fluid produced in the middle ear usually drains down a tube that leads to the throat. This is called the Eustachian tube. If the Eustachian tube becomes blocked by an infection or enlarged adenoids, infected fluid collects in the middle ear. The fluid may become thick and sticky so this problem is also called "glue ear." The "glue" makes it harder for the eardrum and the bones in the middle ear to vibrate properly.

The Eustachian tube lets air from outside into the middle ear. This keeps the air pressure the same on both sides of the eardrum. A blocked Eustachian tube causes air pressure to build up inside the ear. This pressure may damage the eardrum.

## Damaged eardrum

If a person has several serious infections in the middle ear, the eardrum becomes weaker. Eventually, holes or perforations may appear in it. The holes stop the eardrum from vibrating normally and lead to a loss of hearing. Holes in the eardrum usually heal naturally, but if the infection is serious and goes on for a long time, the holes may stay open. This may need special repair treatment. (The medical name for this condition is *chronic otitis media*).

Holes in the eardrum may also be caused by poking things into the ear, a serious blow to the ear, or very loud noises, such as explosions.

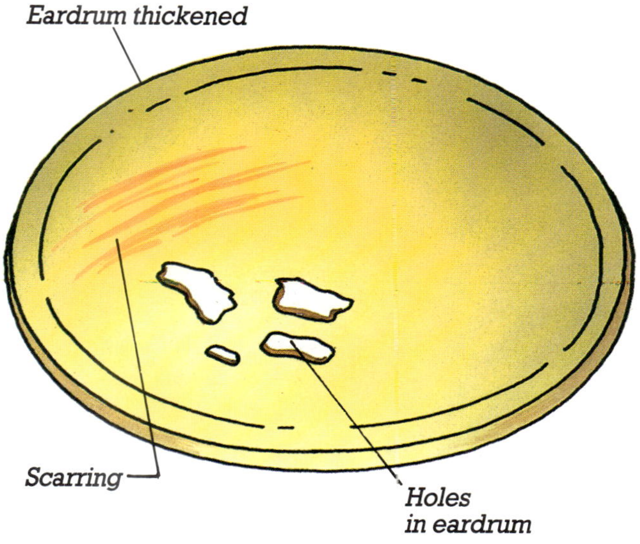


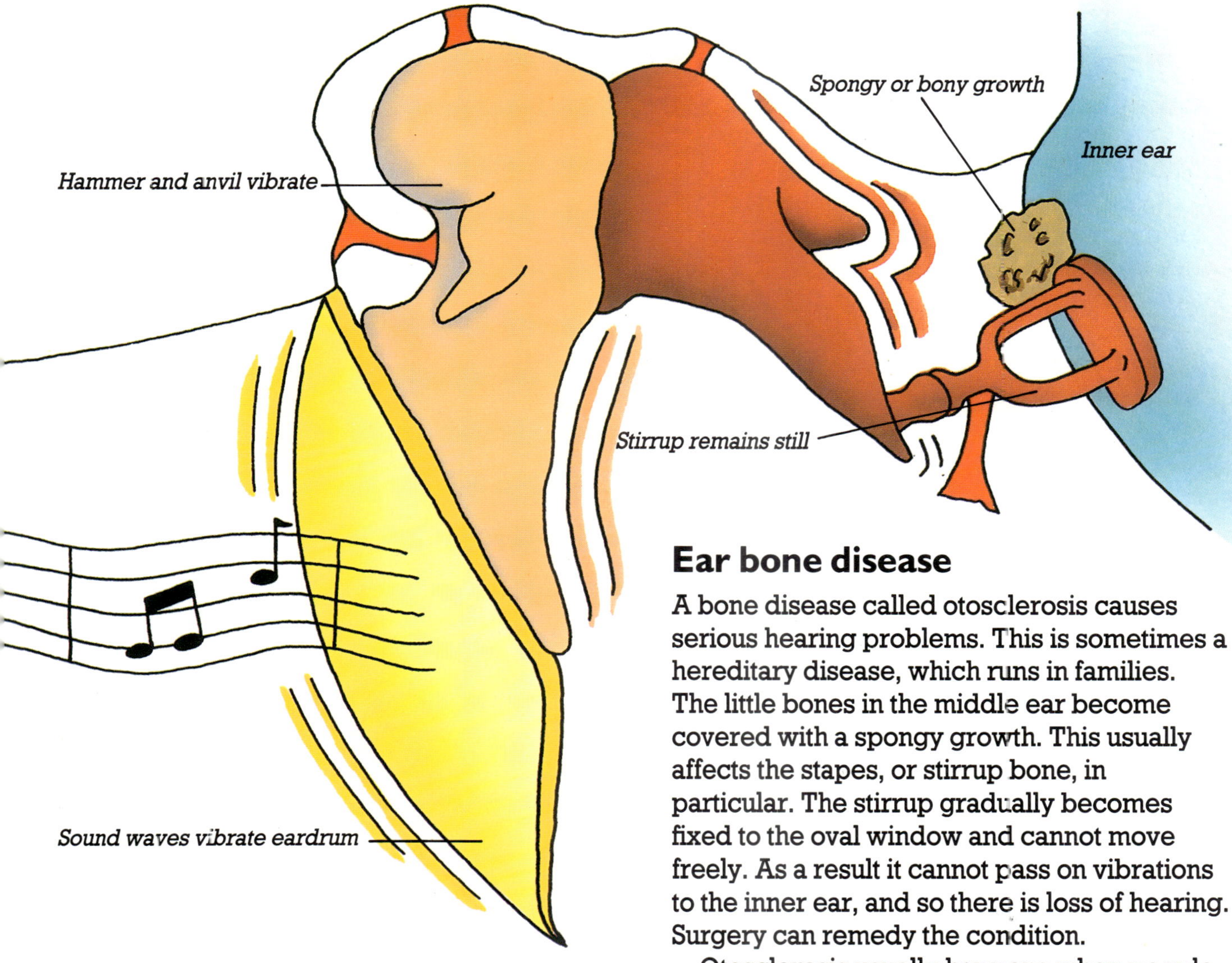


## Ear bone disease

A bone disease called otosclerosis causes serious hearing problems. This is sometimes a hereditary disease, which runs in families. The little bones in the middle ear become covered with a spongy growth. This usually affects the stapes, or stirrup bone, in particular. The stirrup gradually becomes fixed to the oval window and cannot move freely. As a result it cannot pass on vibrations to the inner ear, and so there is loss of hearing. Surgery can remedy the condition.

Otosclerosis usually happens when people are between the ages of 18 and 30, and tends to become more serious as people become older. It is more common in women.

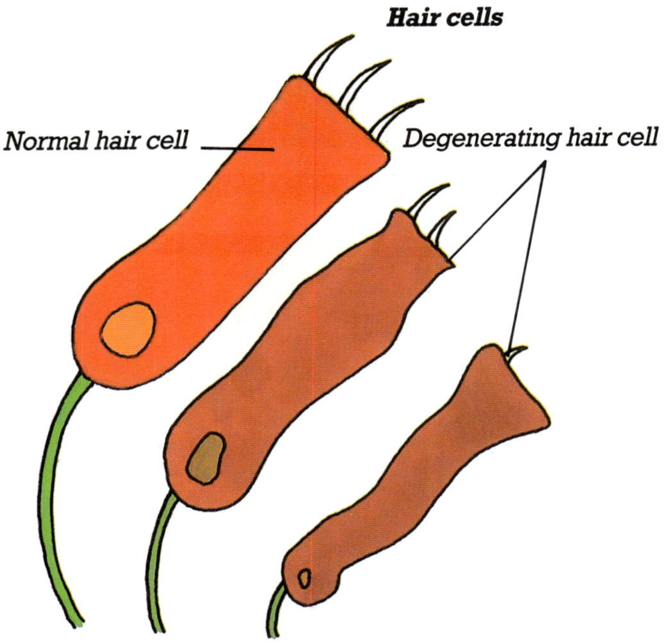


## Nerve deafness

Nerve deafness may develop at any time from before birth through old age. The cochlea is a very sensitive organ and can be damaged by genetic factors, childhood diseases, very loud noises and some drugs. Most elderly people have some form of nerve deafness.

A difficult or premature birth, particularly when the baby does not receive enough oxygen, can cause nerve deafness. Scientists do not understand how this happens. At birth, a baby may develop jaundice, which can damage the auditory nerve and lead to hearing loss. Jaundice is more likely in premature babies. Many of the problems that may occur during birth are becoming less common as better techniques are developed for caring for "at risk" babies.

## Tinnitus

Buzzing or ringing noises in the ears – called tinnitus – affect many people, although the reason for the noises is not clearly understood. It is often hard for a person to determine where in the hearing system the noises are coming from. Some people find the noises almost unbearable. It often occurs in elderly people.

Tinnitus may be caused by very loud noise as well as infections and diseases of the ear. Some people feel that certain drugs and some kinds of food and drink seem to make the noises more unbearable. A person can experience tinnitus without deafness and it can be painful at times.

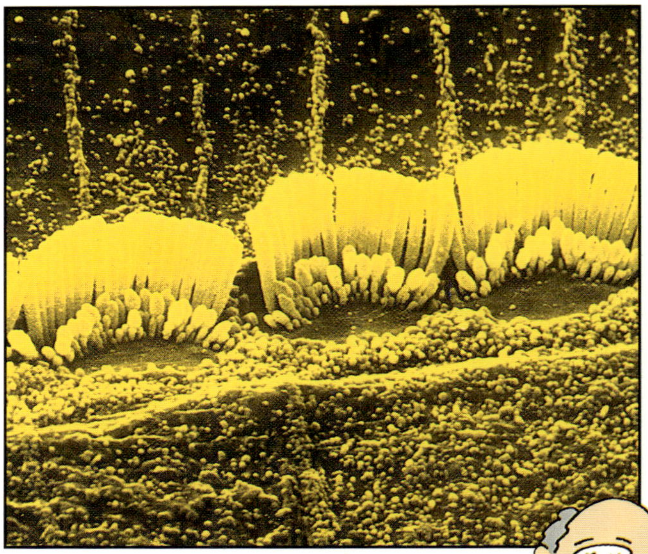

*A row of hair cells in the inner ear*

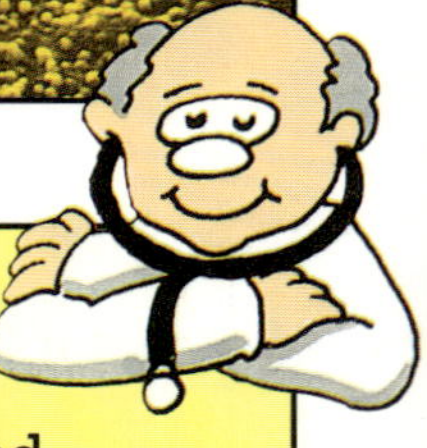

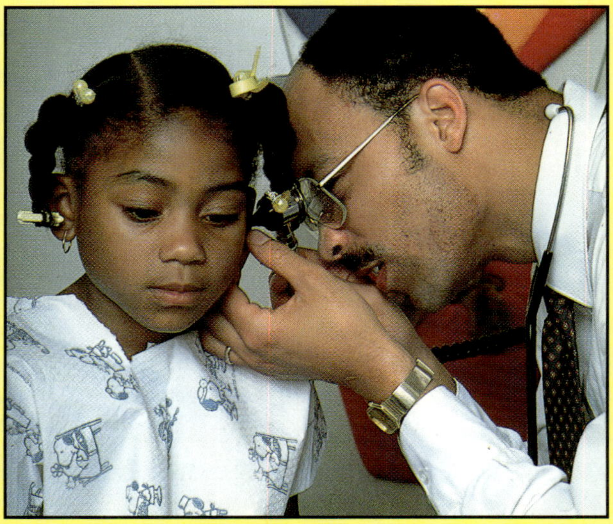

## AN EAR EXAMINATION

A doctor can look into the outer ear and the eardrum with an instrument called an otoscope. With an otoscope a doctor can see if there is a blockage in the ear canal. He or she can also examine the eardrum to see if there are any holes in the surface or if the eardrum is swollen and out of shape. An infection in the middle ear makes the eardrum bulge outward and look red and sore. A surgeon who specializes in problems of the ear is an otologist.

## CHILDHOOD DISEASES

Diseases in childhood may cause severe hearing loss. They include viral diseases such as measles and mumps as well as meningitis, typhoid fever and diphtheria. Any hearing loss tends to occur suddenly at the time of the disease.

Fortunately, only a small number of the people who have these diseases develop a hearing problem. The mumps virus is unusual because it almost always affects one ear only. The other ear remains perfectly normal. The rubella measles virus can affect the developing ears of a baby in the uterus.

A problem only occurs if a bacterial infection damages the cochlea or if a viral infection attacks the hearing nerve.

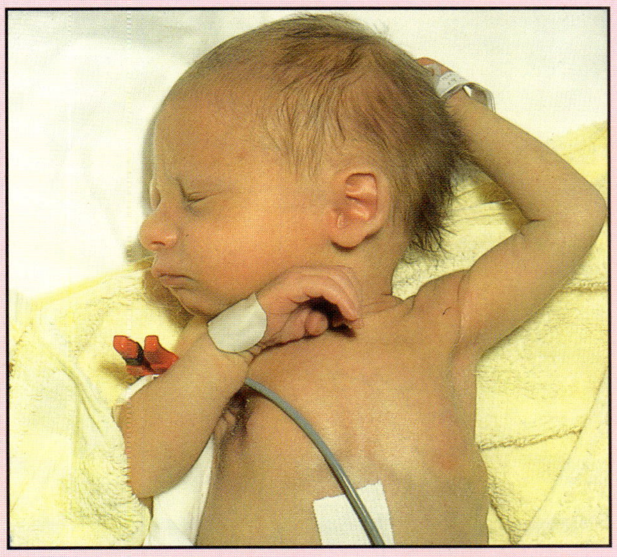

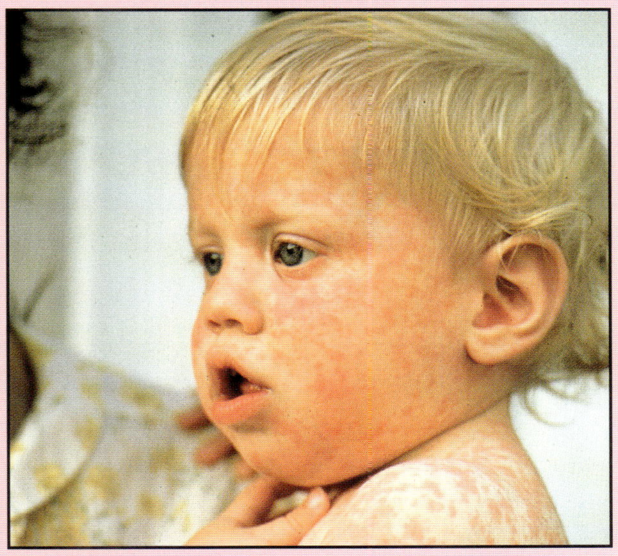

### Meningitis

Meningitis causes the membrane covering the brain to become inflamed. If the infection reaches the throat, nose and ears it may destroy the organ of Corti, in the inner ear, and the auditory nerve.

### Measles

Measles may lead to an infection in the middle ear, or the virus may damage the cochlea. The measles vaccine prevents not only the disease, but its possibly serious consequences as well.

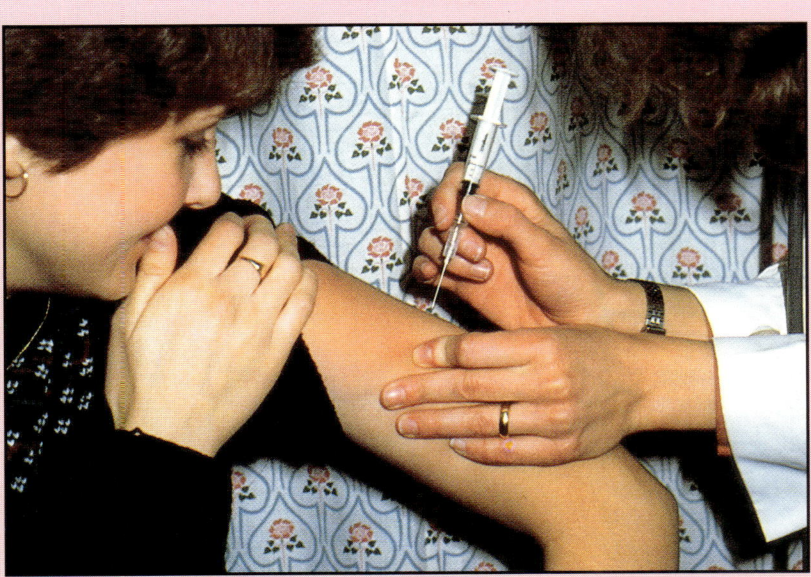

*Girl being given a rubella vaccination*

### Vaccinations

If a woman has rubella for the first time during pregnancy, part of the baby's cochlea may be destroyed. Her baby will be born with nerve deafness. The risks are greatest in the first three months of pregnancy. Fortunately, there are now vaccines that give children protection against rubella, mumps and measles. Most children receive these before the age of two.

# TREATMENT FOR EAR PROBLEMS

Hearing loss in the outer or middle ear can be treated with drugs. Surgery may sometimes be necessary to repair holes in the eardrum or drain infected fluid out of the middle ear. Bone diseases can be treated by replacing the stapes (or stirrup) bone with an artificial one.

It is impossible to cure nerve deafness in the inner ear. But adults or older people, rather than children, can have a cochlear implant. This is a sophisticated hearing aid in which tiny electrodes are implanted in or on the cochlea. This kind of operation relies on the memory of sound and may improve hearing for some people who are almost totally deaf.

Hearing aids make sounds louder, helping the deaf cope with life at home, at school or at work. Hearing aids are worn on the body or behind the ear (these are called post-aural aids). Radio aids provide a direct link from one person to another.

## Detecting deafness in babies

It is difficult to test the hearing of a newborn baby because babies can only respond in a limited way and the responses vary. But a device called an auditory cradle can measure a baby's breathing pattern in response to sound (top right). This does not measure hearing levels or show where a problem is. But, it does indicate possible problems so the baby can be watched carefully and any hearing impediment can be treated.

All babies should have their hearing tested when they are between six and nine months old (lower right). At this age, they can hold up their heads without help. If they hear a sound which is made behind them, they are able to turn towards the sound. This is called distraction testing. The tester makes the sounds at a low level at first but, if the baby does not turn round, the level is increased until he or she responds.

Ear infections are a very common condition in babies and toddlers who may not even complain of earache but simply feel unwell, with perhaps a temperature. For this reason doctors always examine the ears of young children who have a fever.

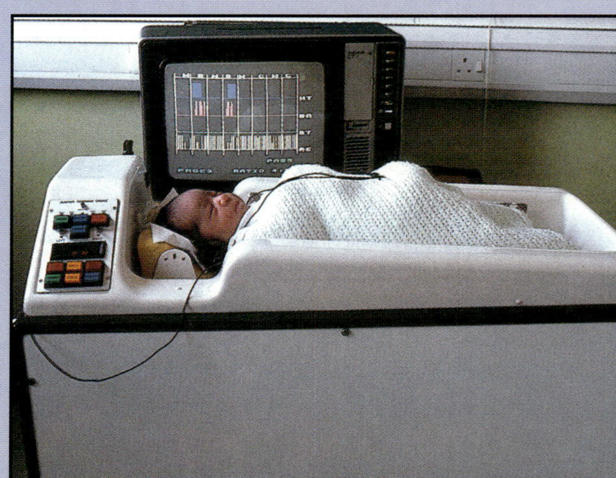

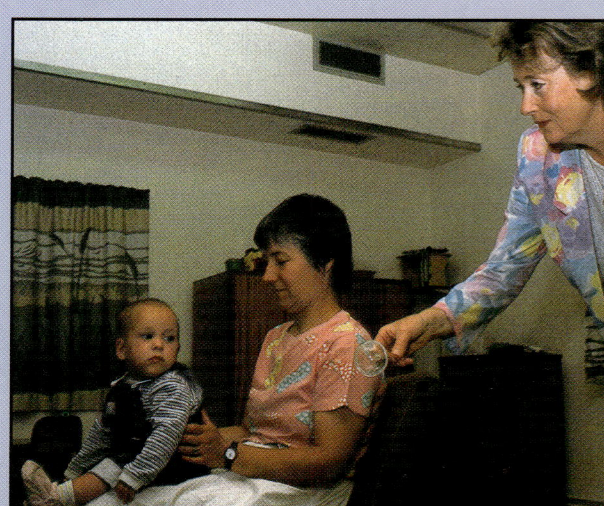

## Hearing tests

Older children can take more part in hearing tests. They play special games that make use of their understanding of speech. The tester may give the child a toy and ask the child to "put it in the box" or "give it to Mommy." The levels of sound used in these games are measured with a meter. This helps the tester to discover the most quiet sounds that a child can hear.

At the age of about two years, children can be given a performance test. In this test, the child is asked to put small wooden pieces into a wooden board when the tester says "go." This tests low frequency sounds. A similar test using a hissing sound tests high frequency.

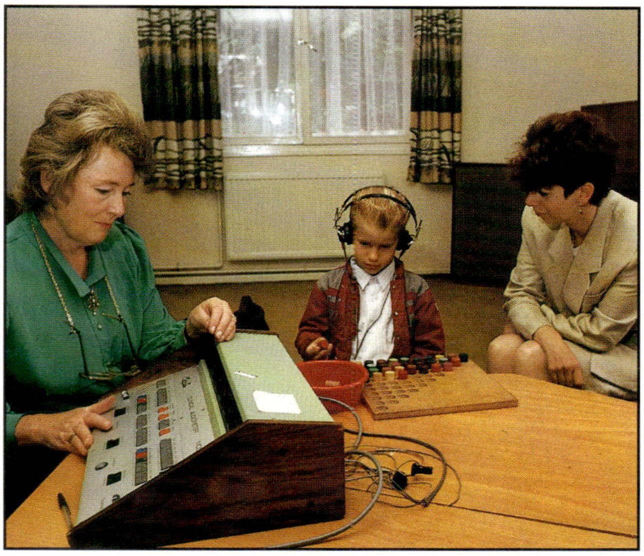

*A performance test*

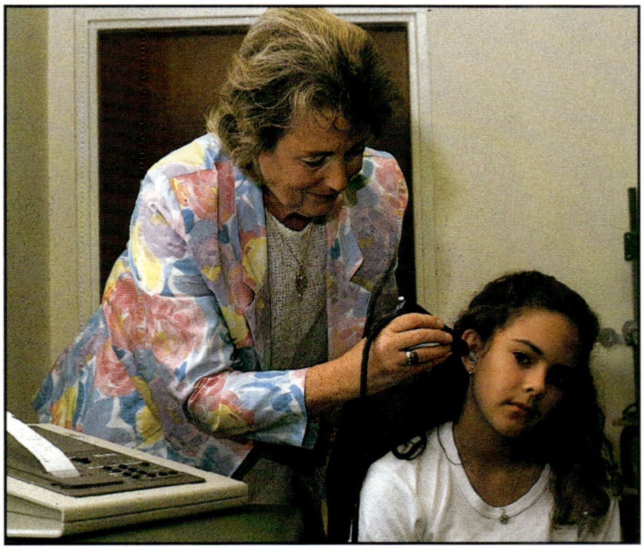

*An audiometer measures tones*

## Pure tone audiometry

From the age of about three years onwards, it is possible to measure hearing more precisely with a test called pure tone audiometry. The person listens through headphones to a series of tones produced by a machine called an audiometer (left). Each tone is a different frequency (pitch). The loudness of the tone is reduced until the person can just hear it.

The results of the test are plotted on a chart called an audiogram. This shows the frequency and loudness of the sounds the person was able to hear. The results for the right ear are plotted as small circles. For the left ear, the results are plotted as crosses.

## An Artificial ear

Some babies are born with no ears, and to remedy this condition artificial ears with a special titanium hearing aid implant can be made. First a titanium hearing aid is implanted and integrated into the bone tissue and then the new ear is fitted. The ears look real and allow the patient to feel more confident, wear glasses, swim, play sports and be more easily accepted at school.

In other cases, perhaps after the ear has been badly damaged in an accident, plastic surgery may help. The surgeon uses skin from other parts of the body to reconstruct a replacement outer ear, which allows the hearing system to work as normally as possible.

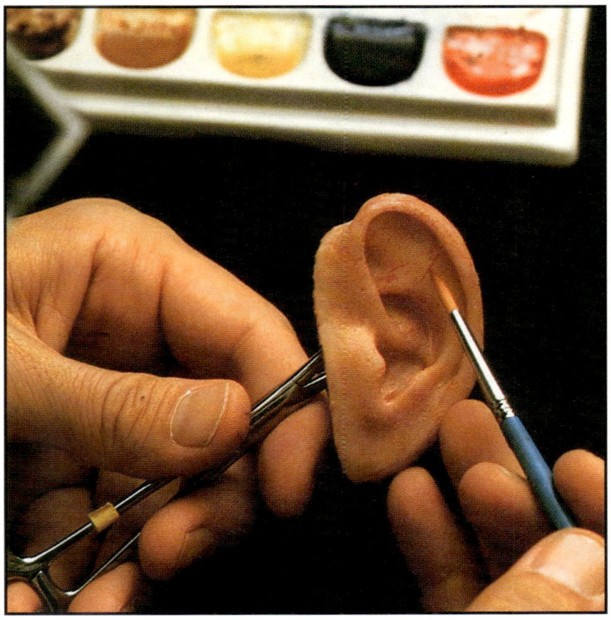

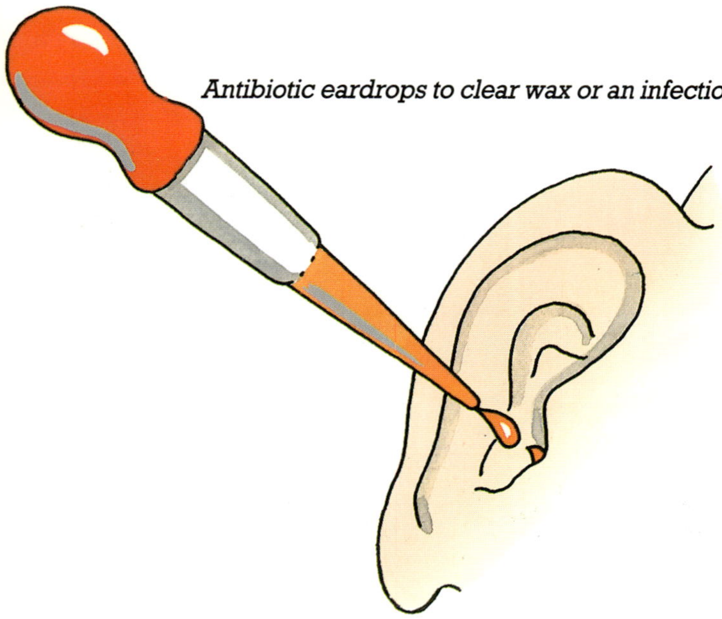

*Antibiotic eardrops to clear wax or an infection*

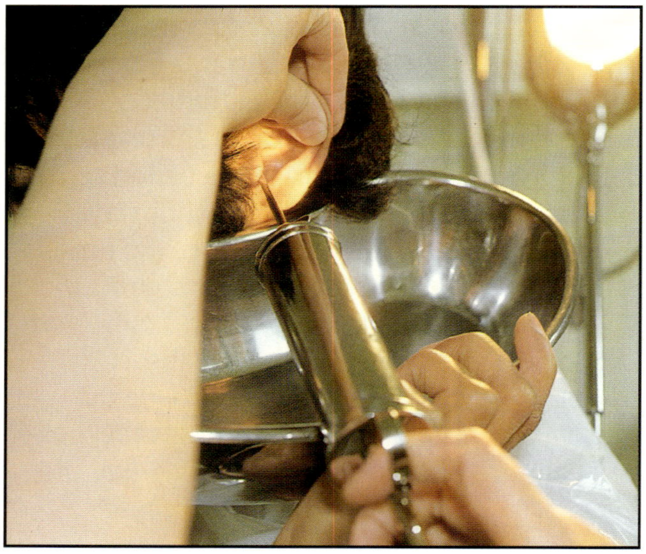

*A doctor washing an ear canal with a syringe*

## Outer ear treatments

If there is too much wax in the ear canal and the wax has become hardened, it may not be able to move out of the ear naturally. It is best to ask a doctor about kinds of eardrops or other remedies, because they may cause allergic reactions in some people. If the wax continues to be a problem, a doctor can remove it by using a syringe to wash it out. But if syringing is carried out too often, it seems to reduce the natural process of wax movement. So, after a time, syringing has to be carried out more and more frequently.

It is not easy to treat an infection in the ear canal, and it is important to treat it before it becomes too serious. An ear infection is more likely to clear up quickly if you consult a doctor as soon as possible. The other important point is to keep the ear dry at all times, so that antibiotic eardrops can be used to try and combat the infection. As with drops that are used to clear wax, some people may be allergic to antibiotic drops.

If a person is born with no ears or only rudimentary ears, or no ear canal, surgeons may be able to operate and try to correct the defect. Operations to create an ear canal are difficult and do not usually restore hearing to a useful level. But the surgeon may be able to make an ear canal that is large enough to take a hearing aid, making it a worthwhile operation.

## Sealing holes in the eardrum

Occasionally, holes in the eardrum do not heal (right). If this happens, an operation can remedy the problem. A small piece of muscle is joined over the hole, and this grows onto the eardrum to seal it.

If the perforation is too large for this kind of surgery, a whole eardrum can be transplanted. Artificial eardrums may also be used.

A "popping" sound in the ears when we descend rapidly in an elevator is caused by small movements of the eardrum through changes of pressure in the middle ear. This kind of pressure change is not dangerous and will not normally damage the eardrum.

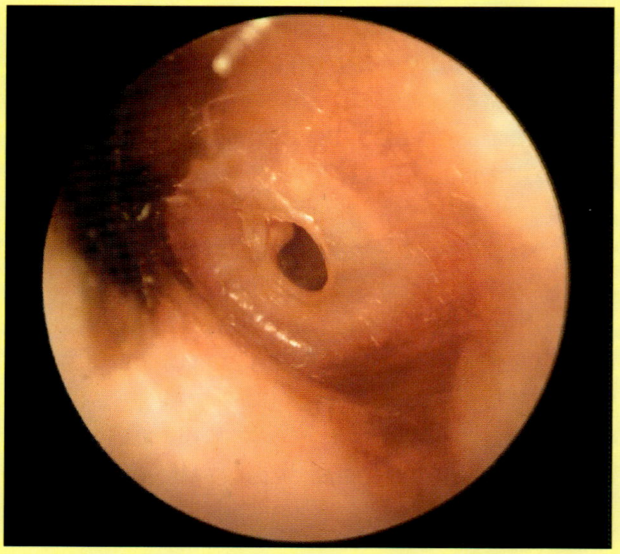

## Mastoid surgery

If infections in the middle ear are not cleared up with antibiotics, the infection can spread to the ear bones. Over a long period of time, the infection may even spread to the mastoid bone behind the ear. Once this happens, the bone or part of the bone has to be removed. The middle ear bones may also have to be removed, so this operation does not usually improve hearing. If a cavity is left in the mastoid bone, wax and other debris may collect so the cavity has to be cleaned out from time to time. Mastoid operations are less common nowadays.

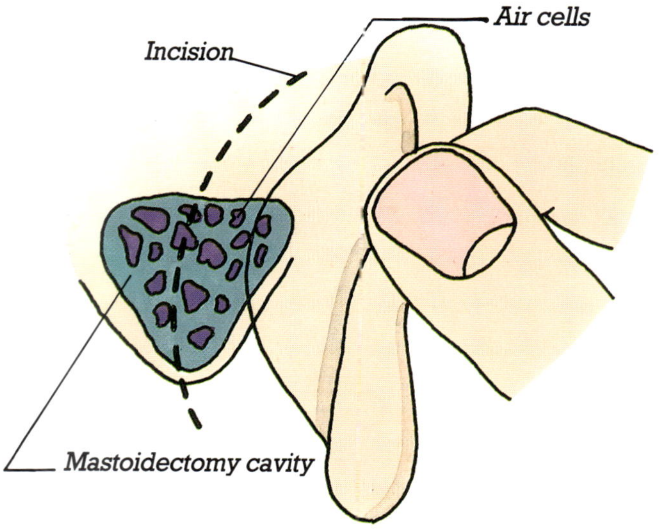


## Grommets

If there is a buildup of fluid in the middle ear, a tiny slit in the eardrum can be made and the infected fluid "sucked out." Sometimes, after the operation a small plastic tube called a grommet, or ventilation tube, is pushed through the slit. This stays in place for up to a year, and allows any more excess fluid to drain away. The grommet eventually falls out of the eardrum and comes out of the ear on its own. The slit in the eardrum usually heals naturally.

Grommets are often inserted when young children suffer with a series of ear infections and the grommet falls out as the ear canal grows and develops naturally as part of the child's development.

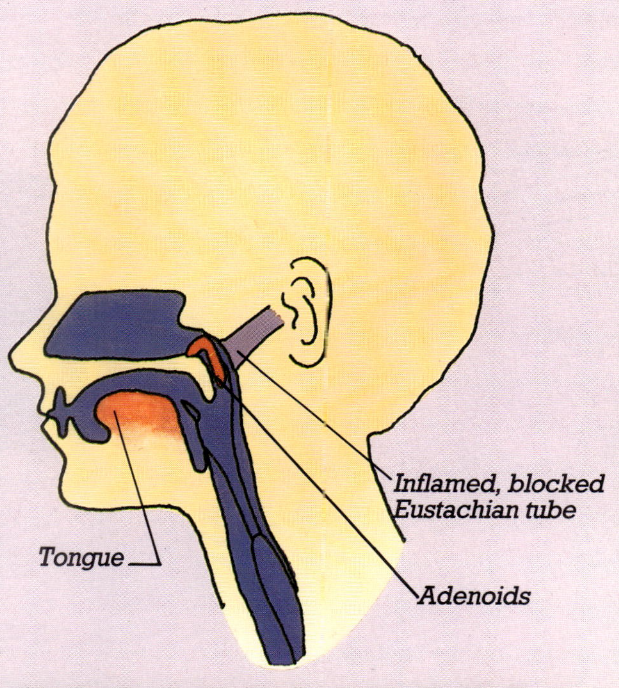


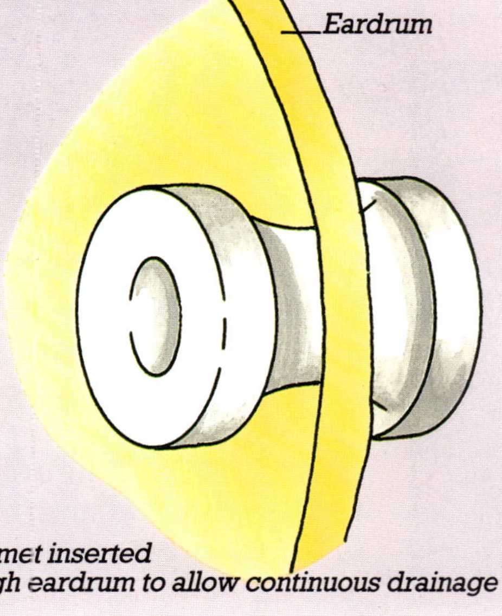


*Grommet inserted through eardrum to allow continuous drainage*

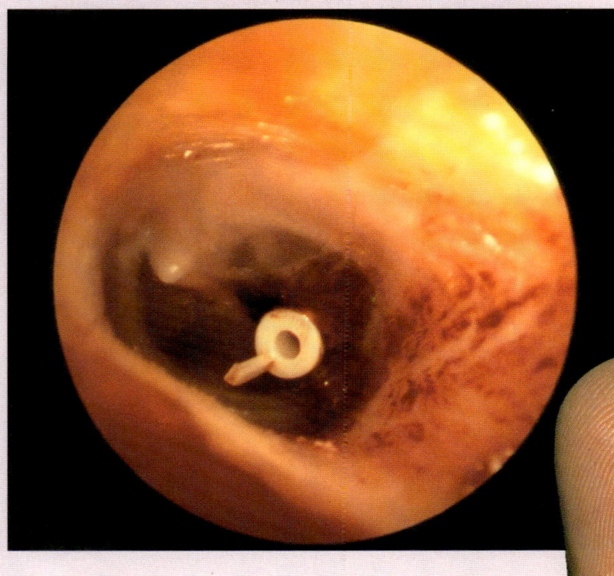

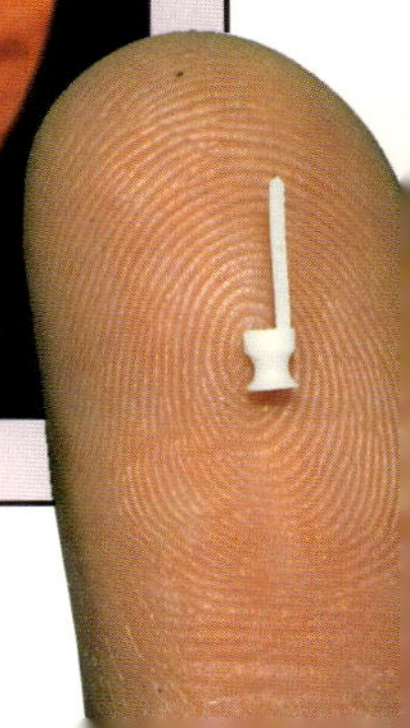

## Surgery for ear bone problems

In the recent past there was little that doctors could do to help people with problems in the inner part of their ear. But with modern surgical techniques this situation has drastically changed. The disease in which a bony growth stops the middle ear bones from vibrating freely, called otosclerosis, affects many people. The symptoms include a gradual decrease in hearing, sometimes accompanied by tinnitus. In the first stages of the disease a hearing aid can help the person to hear. But as time goes on, the disease progresses and a hearing aid is no longer useful. For this reason, and because people often suffer from this condition at an early age, surgery is usually carried out.

The original operation to remedy the problem was called a fenestration operation. A hole is made in the mastoid bone behind the ear. Sound waves can then bypass the middle ear by traveling through the hole directly to the cochlea in the inner ear. This operation, though effective has now been replaced by an operation called a stapedectomy, which give a better chance of the person hearing almost normally again.

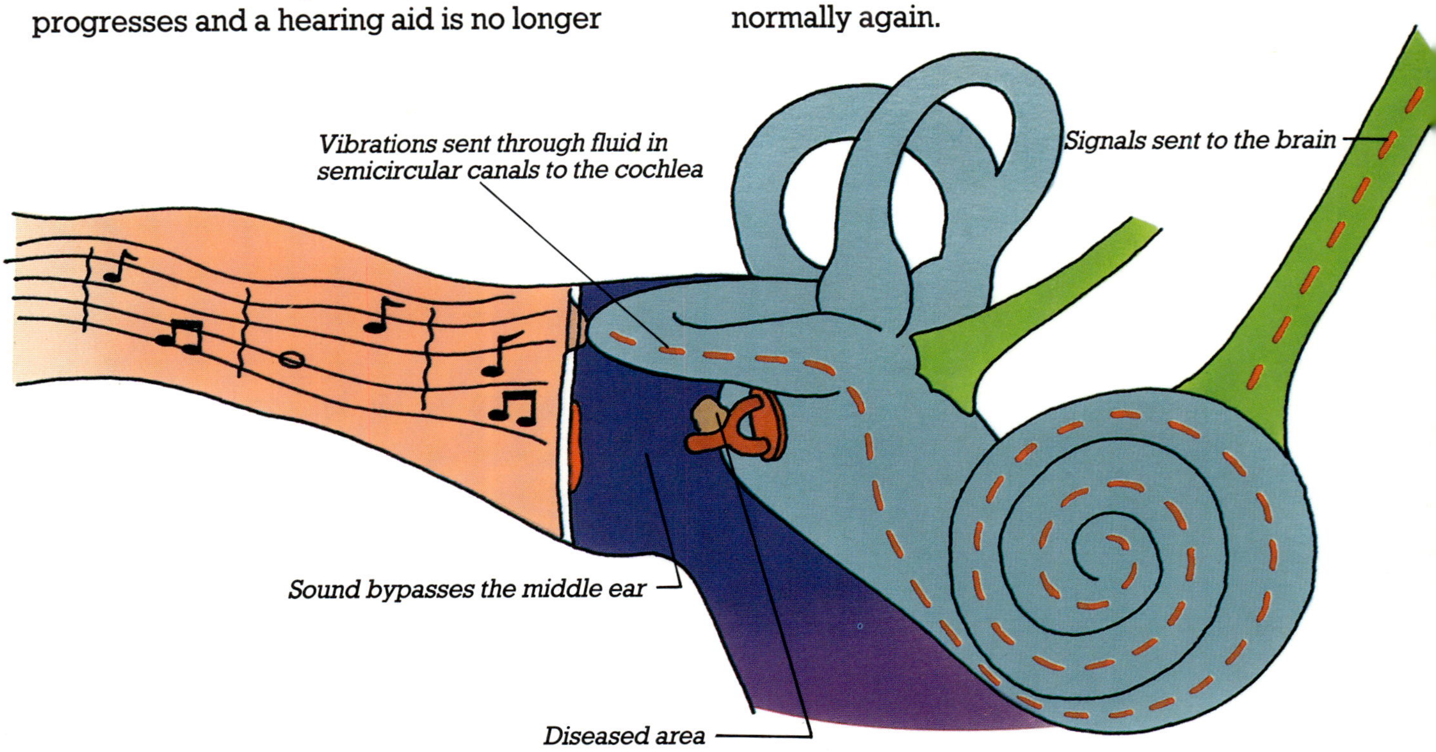


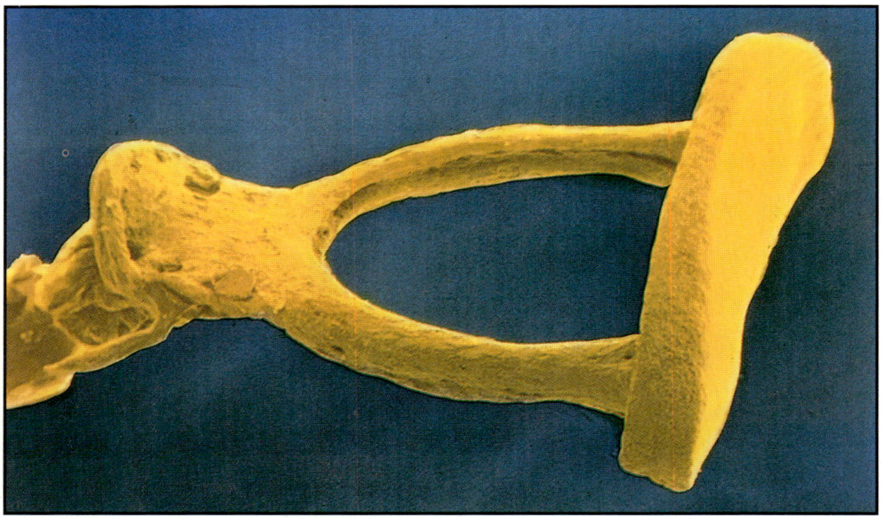
Electron micrograph of a stirrup bone

## Stapedectomy

A stapedectomy operation is carried out to remove the stapes (stirrup) bone in the middle ear and replace it with a metal or plastic one. If the operation is not carried out when the ear is affected by otosclerosis, bony growth eventually stops the stapes from vibrating against the oval window. As a result, vibrations do not reach the cochlea in the inner ear.

## Cochlear implants

Cochlear implants are minute hearing aids, which are powered by batteries, worn in a speech synthesizer box. During surgery, a tiny electrode is placed on or inside the cochlea in the inner ear. The electrode is designed to carry an electric current which stimulates the nerve endings in the cochlea.

The current for the electrode comes from an electronic box strapped onto a person's body. This processes the sound picked up by a microphone and passes it to two coils. One coil is behind the ear and the other is under the skin close to the ear. The coils trigger a current in the electrode remotely. They are not connected to the electrode to cut down on the risk of infection.

Cochlear implants divert sound waves straight to the cochlea and can help people who are profoundly deaf. But, they can only help a person to recognize sounds, and so are not a cure for deafness.

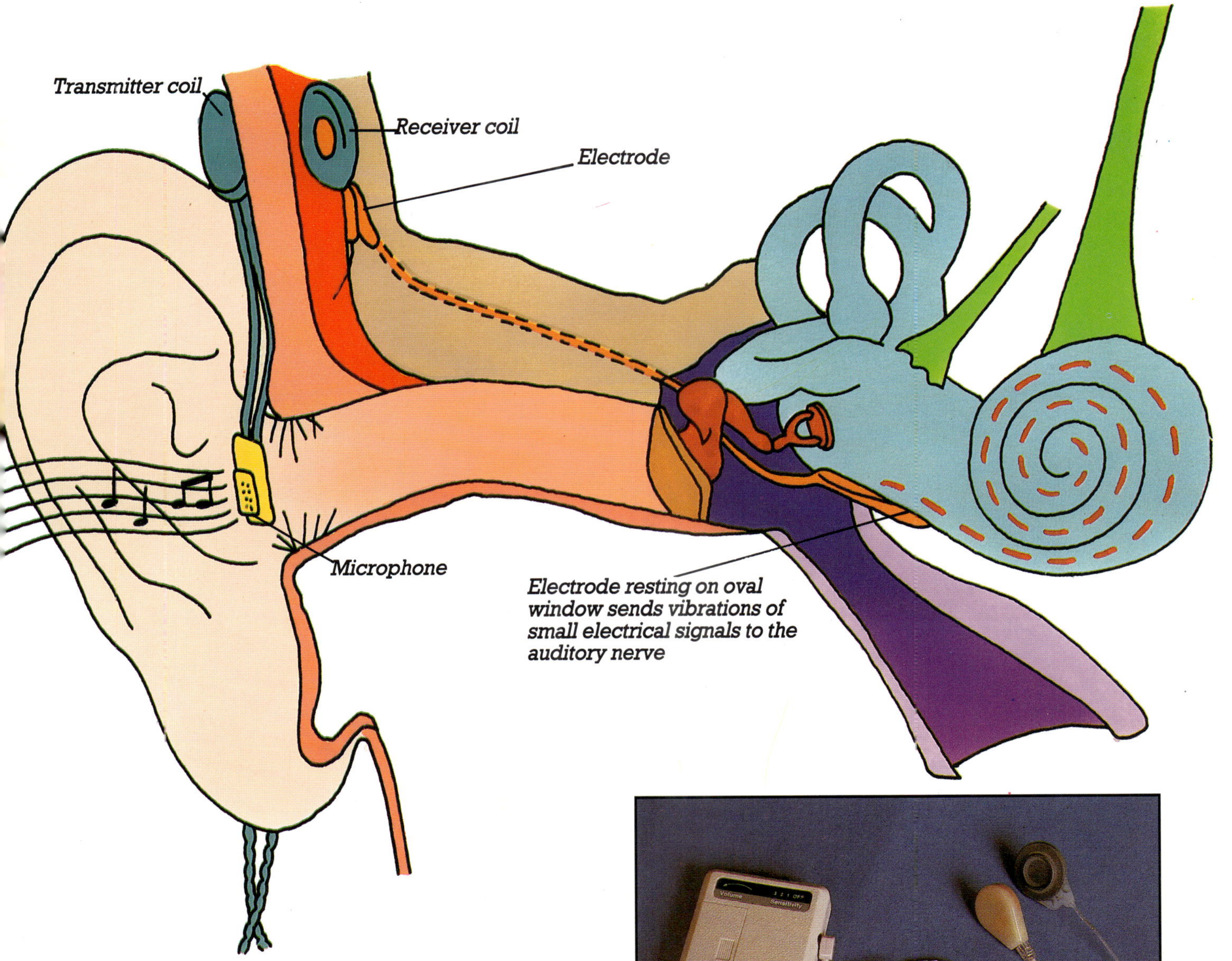


As cochlear implants rely on the memory of sound, there have been very few of these operations performed on children. World wide, about 3,000 people have received cochlear implants. The diagnosis of deafness is not accurate enough in very young children to justify using cochlear implants.

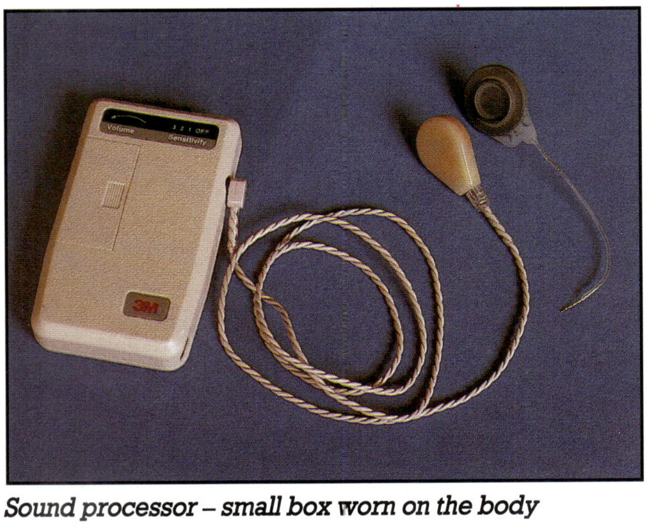

*Sound processor – small box worn on the body*

## Hearing aids

A hearing aid is designed to pick up sounds and make them louder. It does not make the sounds clearer. Hearing aids that are carried on the body usually make sounds louder than those that are worn behind the ear.

One of the problems with hearing aids is that the batteries need to be replaced frequently, sometimes as often as three times a week. The battery for early hearing aids used to be very large and cumbersome. Fortunately, modern hearing aids have much smaller batteries. Some fit snugly behind the ear in a miniaturized unit and are only about the size of a shirt button. The earmold part of the aid fits inside the ear and feeds sound from the hearing aid down the ear canal to the eardrum. Earmolds are made from an impression taken of the ear with a soft rubbery substance.

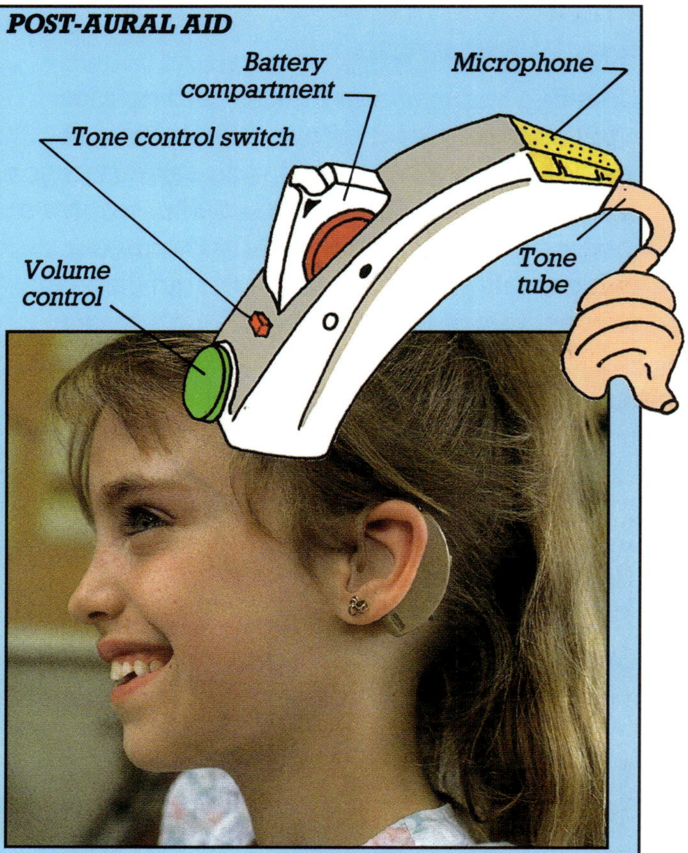

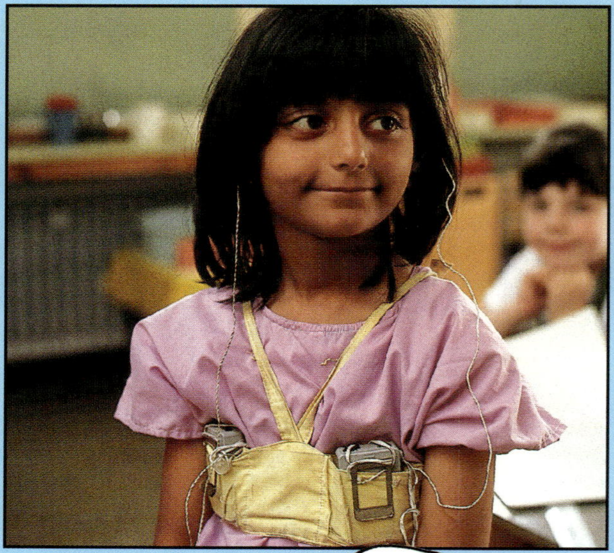

## Loop systems

Loop systems are used in public places, such as theaters (their logo is shown here). They can even be built into a telephone earpiece. A wire loop is connected to the source of a sound, such as a television set.

The wire gives out a magnetic field. This can be picked up by a hearing aid, which converts the magnetic field back into sound. The loop system cuts out background noises and echoes.

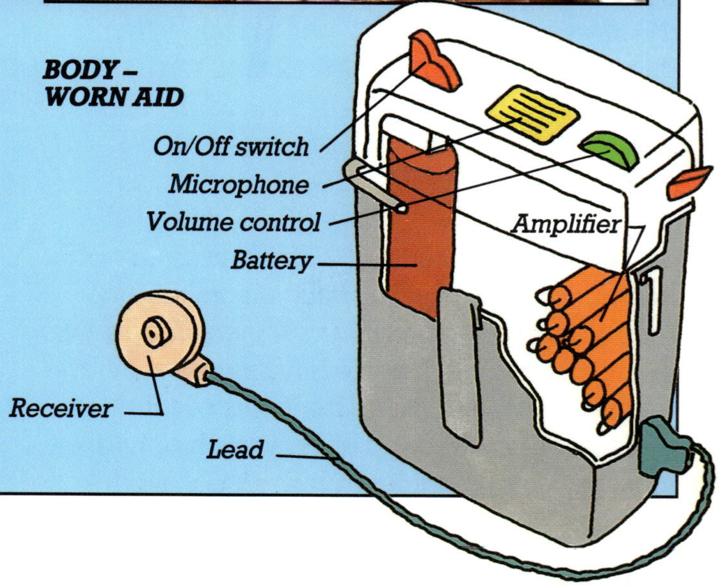

## Radio aids in the classroom

There are often many background noises in a classroom, and this can make it hard for the child to hear what the teacher is saying with an ordinary hearing aid. Sound waves become weaker as they travel through air. Radio aids overcome this problem by using radio waves, which do not lose as much strength as sound waves do when they travel through air. Radio aids are very expensive though, and need to have their batteries charged every night.

Radio aids send sounds directly from one person to another. They are made up of two parts. The teacher wears a radio transmitter linked to a microphone. Radio waves from the transmitter are picked up by a radio receiver, which the child wears. The receiver may also work as a hearing aid and pass louder sounds to the child's ears. Or the receiver may pass the signals on to the child's ordinary hearing aid. In a school, each class may need its own separate frequency or wavelength to tune into, so that a child in one class does not pick up signals from another class.

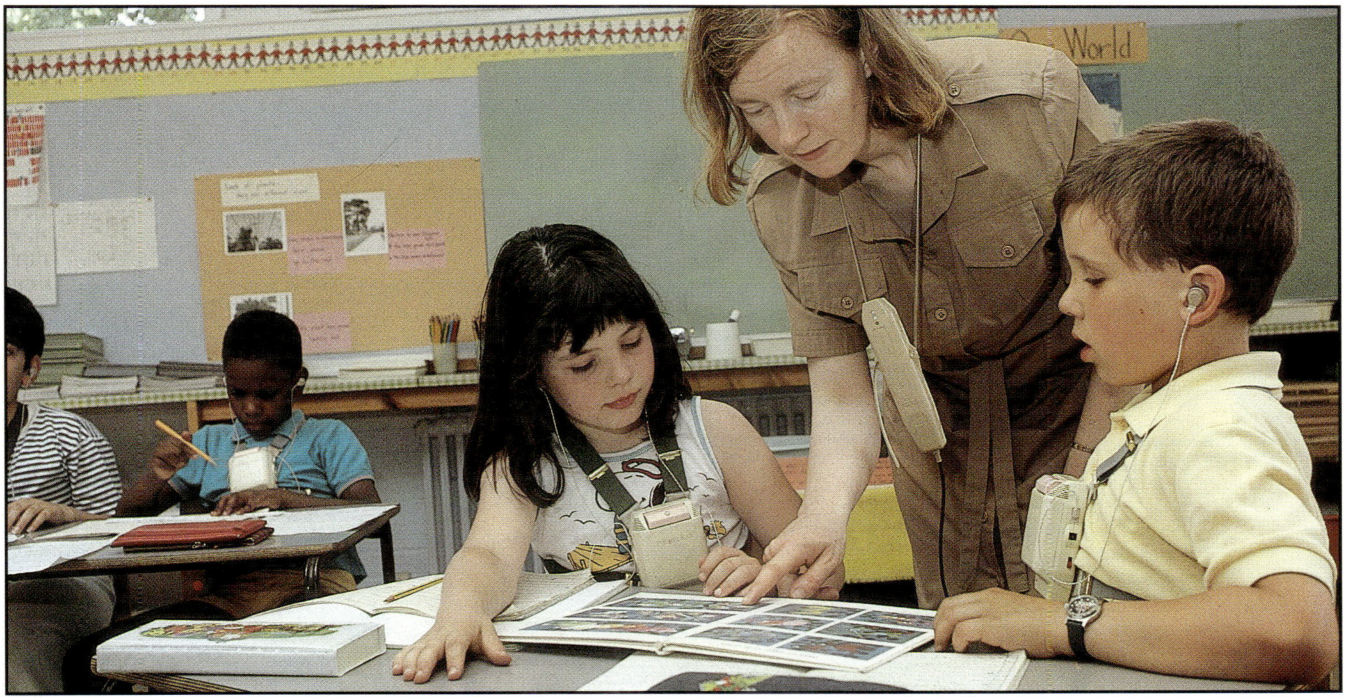


*Radiophonic aid being used in a classroom*

## Tinnitus masker

Small machines that look like hearing aids may help people who suffer from tinnitus (right). These machines are called maskers because they make a gentle, rushing sound that "masks" or covers up the uncomfortable buzzing or ringing noises. The masker is most useful if it makes noises at the same loudness and frequency as the noises in the person's ears or head. It is often very difficult to determine which are the problem frequencies for a particular person. This is because the noises are something that only the person can hear. Tinnitus maskers also boost sounds from outside the head which makes the sufferer less aware of the tinnitus. But some people simply have to learn to live with tinnitus.

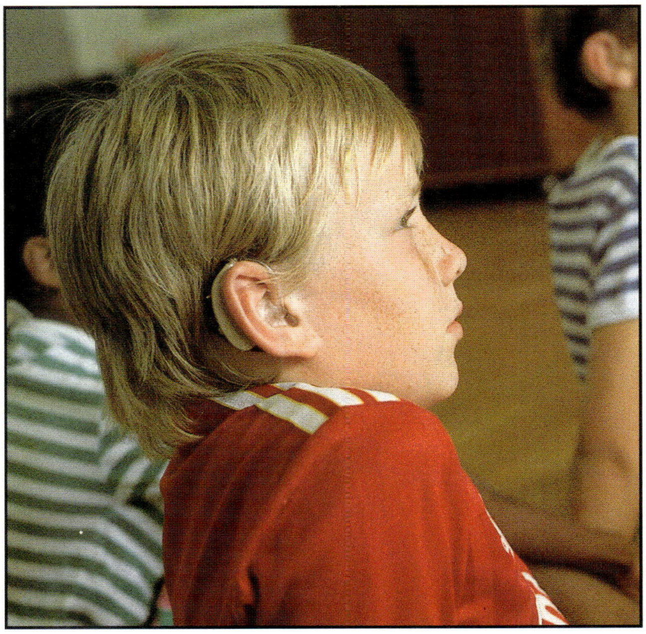

# LIVING WITH DEAFNESS

If a person finds it hard or even impossible to hear, it is more difficult to cope with everyday life, education, work and leisure activities. The kinds of difficulties depend on the type and amount of deafness. For example, some people cannot hear high frequency sounds, and so cannot hear consonants such as "s," "t," and "th" or "sh" in speech. People born with a hearing loss find it very difficult to learn how to speak. It is especially important that they are encouraged to use a variety of methods of communication, including sign language and lipreading and to use hearing aids. If people with a hearing loss are given help and encouragement from a very early age there is no reason why they should not do well at school. Many children with a hearing impairment do not go to special schools. With care and understanding, from parents and teachers and other social relationships, children that are hard of hearing can achieve a high standard of education and go to college and pursue all kinds of interesting careers.

## Everyday living

Many everyday events, such as answering the door bell or getting up on time,cause problems for people with a hearing loss. Some electronic devices may make life easier. These include adaptors that make lights flash or special pads that vibrate when bells ring. Some alarm clocks have a pad that fits under the mattress or pillow and vibrates to wake you up. A telephone can have an amplifier or a loop system (see page 18) fitted. The loop system can be linked to a hearing aid. Another device that helps people that are hard of hearing is a viewdata adaptor. Connected to a telephone line it allows a person to see the information from a telephone call written on a television screen. In Great Britain there is a telephone exchange for the deaf where an operator types what the person is saying. The words appear on a screen in the deaf person's home or office. It is perfectly possible for deaf people to lead a normal and useful life. Some authorities allow partially deaf people to drive – provided warning sounds are converted into visual signals.

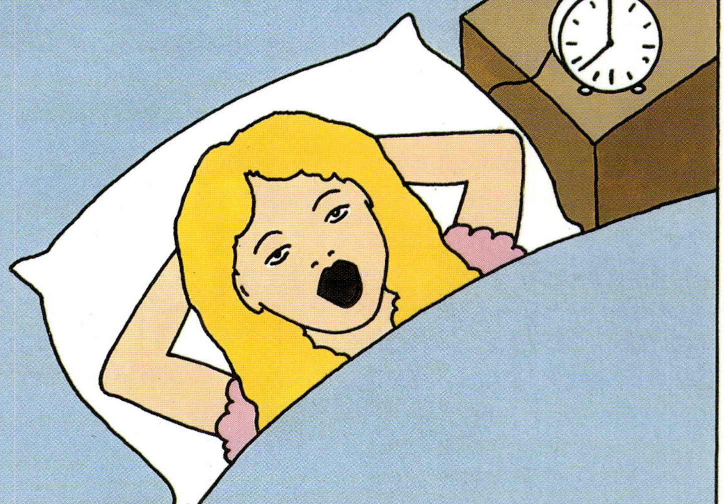

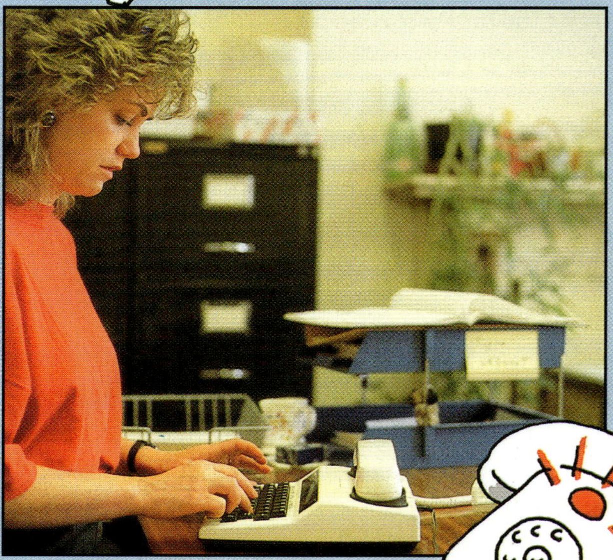

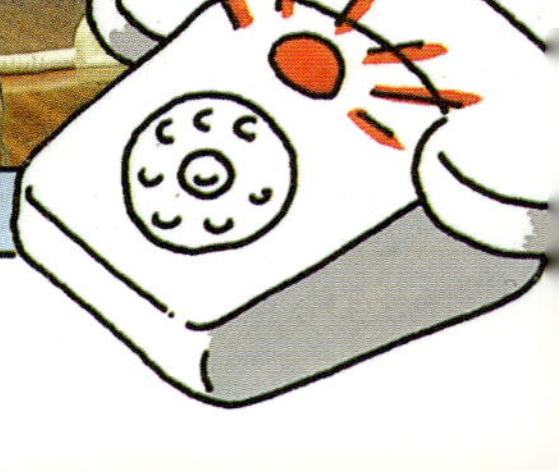

## Visual aids

Television has many advantages for people with hearing problems because it can communicate visually. But listening is also important with television. This is often a major problem for a person with a hearing loss. Turning up the volume is not usually the answer because this may irritate other members of the family or neighbors. In some countries, a small percentage of programs have subtitles or captions and sign language so that deaf people will find the information easier to follow and understand. If subtitles were available on more television programs, it would make it much easier for deaf people to enjoy watching television.

Some television channels show electronic "magazines" of information with words and diagrams on all sorts of topics, such as news, travel, finance and sport. There may be special "magazines" for people with a hearing loss. These may include a summary of a play or drama series which will be appearing on television in the near future or news (above right). This sort of preparation helps deaf people to follow the action more easily. You need a special type of television to receive these magazine programs.

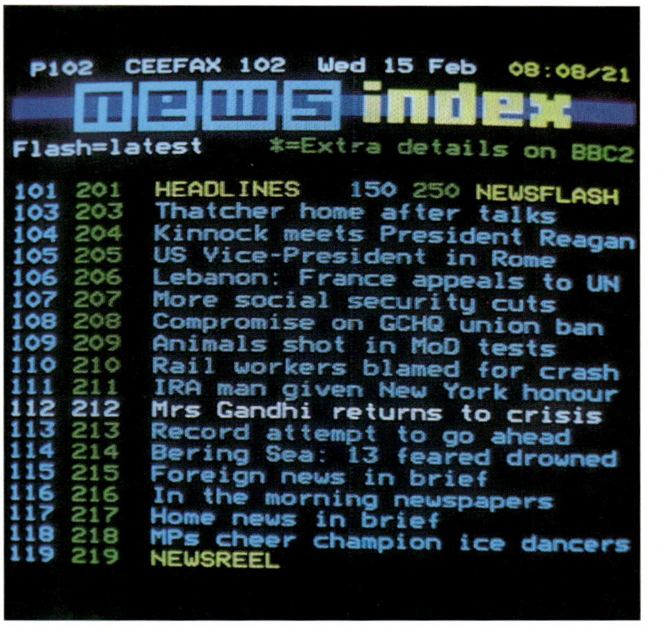
P102 CEEFAX 102 Wed 15 Feb 08:08/21
news index
Flash=latest *=Extra details on BBC2
101 201 HEADLINES 150 250 NEWSFLASH
103 203 Thatcher home after talks
104 204 Kinnock meets President Reagan
105 205 US Vice-President in Rome
106 206 Lebanon: France appeals to UN
107 207 More social security cuts
108 208 Compromise on GCHQ union ban
109 209 Animals shot in MoD tests
110 210 Rail workers blamed for crash
111 211 IRA man given New York honour
112 212 Mrs Gandhi returns to crisis
113 213 Record attempt to go ahead
114 214 Bering Sea: 13 feared drowned
115 215 Foreign news in brief
116 216 In the morning newspapers
117 217 Home news in brief
118 218 MPs cheer champion ice dancers
119 219 NEWSREEL

*Visual news on television*

Many televisions have a socket that takes headphones, a special microphone or an infra-red listening device. You can also have a loop system (see page 18) fitted in the home so you can listen to the television through a hearing aid. With a loop system, you can hear the television as if the sound were coming straight from the loudspeaker. But you will not hear background noise, such as other people talking in the room.

***Television listening devices***

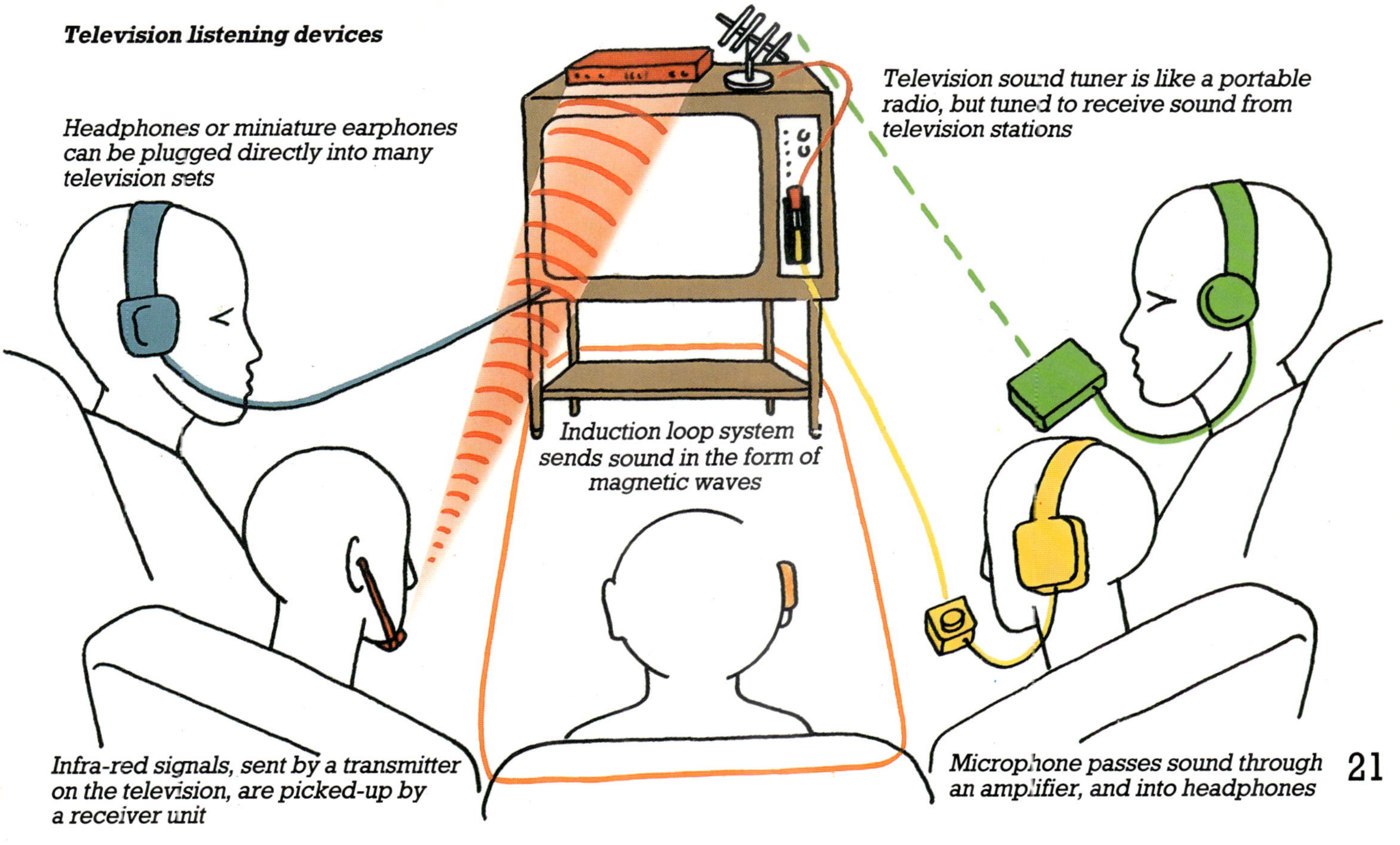

## Fingerspelling and sign language

Fingerspelling is a language that uses hand and finger shapes to represent the letters of the alphabet. This is called a manual alphabet. Throughout the world, there are many types of manual alphabet. Many, such as the United States version, use one hand. This leaves the other hand free for other tasks. Other manual alphabets, such as the British one, use two hands.

With practice, you can learn fingerspelling very quickly. Fingerspelling can be used as a way of communicating by touch with people who are both deaf and blind. Sign language is a different sort of language that uses hand shapes and hand movements as well as eye movements, facial expressions and body positions to stand for whole words or ideas.

*United States fingerspelling*

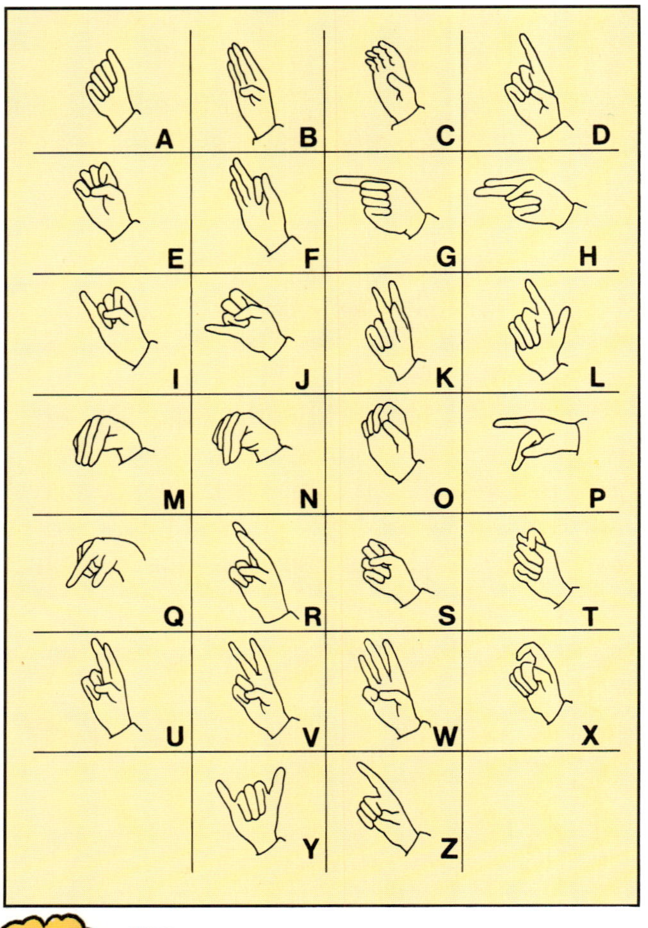


*British fingerspelling*

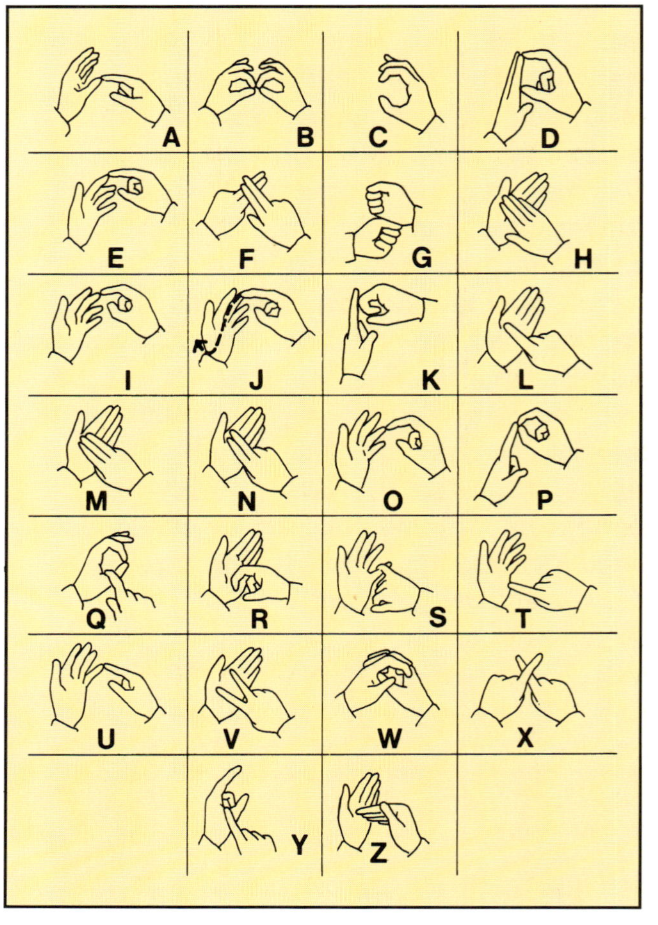


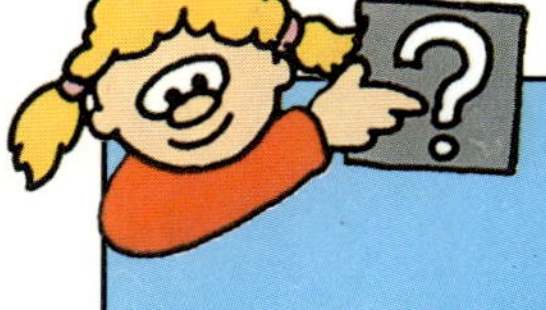


### Signs

Signs for words or ideas are made with the hands but meaning is also given by the expression of the face and position of the body. It takes a long time and much patience to learn how to sign well.

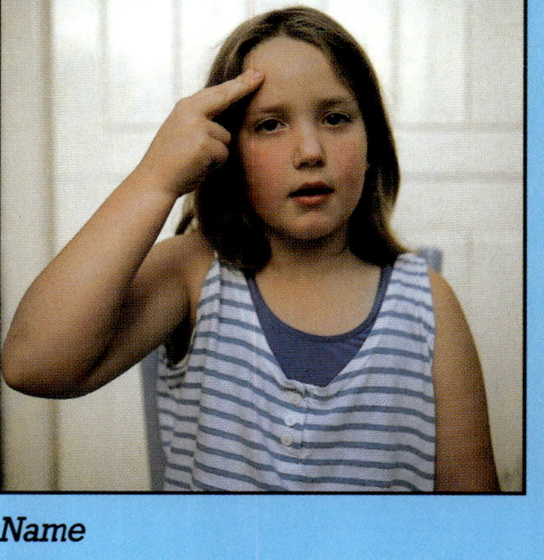

*Name*

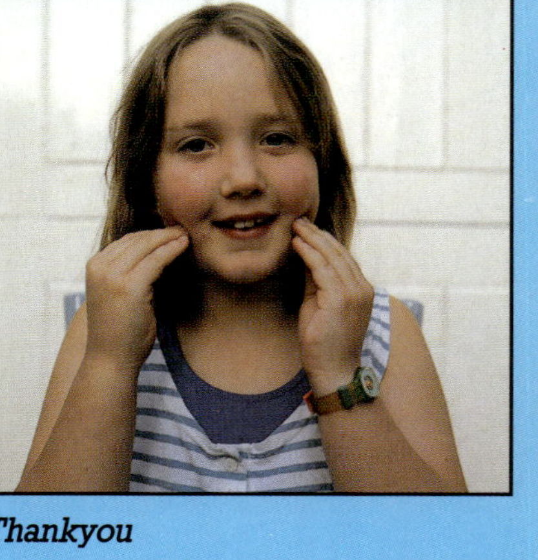

*Thankyou*

## Lipreading or speech reading

A person with a hearing loss may be able to work out the sounds a person is making by "reading" the shape of the lips. This is called lipreading or speech reading. The technique can be of some use if the speaker forms the words clearly. But even the best lipreader probably reads only 50 percent of the words spoken. The rest is just guesswork. Many sounds in the English language are invisible on the lips. For example, the difference between the words "goal" and "coal" depend only on sounds made in the throat. Other sounds, such as "p", "b" and "m", "d" and "n" and "s" and "z" can be easily confused. If you do not know much about the subject of a conversation, lipreading is even more difficult. For a person who has been born deaf, lipreading is much more difficult than for a person who used to be able to hear. This is because a deaf person has to imagine sounds that have never been heard.

Deafness or even a slight difficulty in hearing impairment can lead to a loss of confidence and a feeling of being excluded from everyday living. As a result, deafness can be a considerable social barrier as no one likes being in a situation in which he or she feels ill at ease. Lipreading does not come naturally and must be learned.

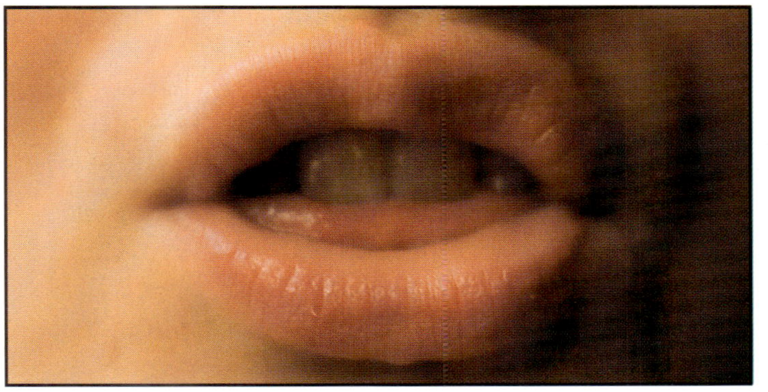

*Lips making an "th" sound*

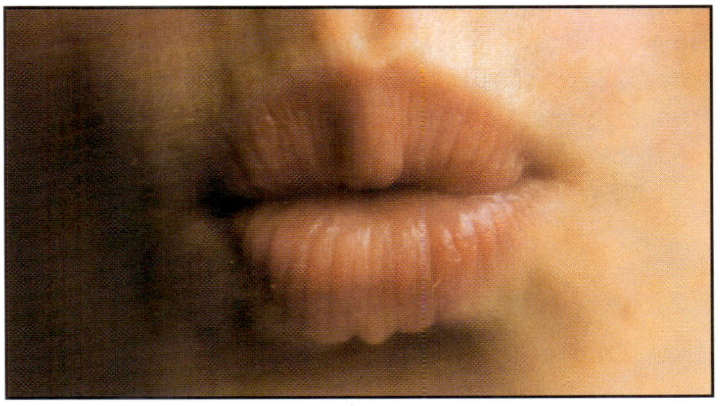

*Lips making an "o" sound*

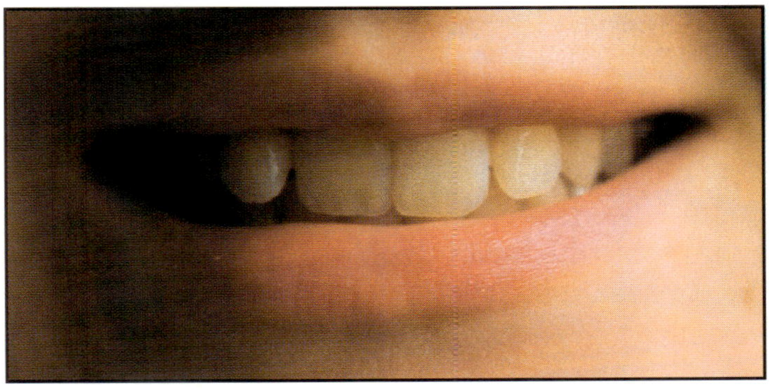

*Lips making a "e" sound*

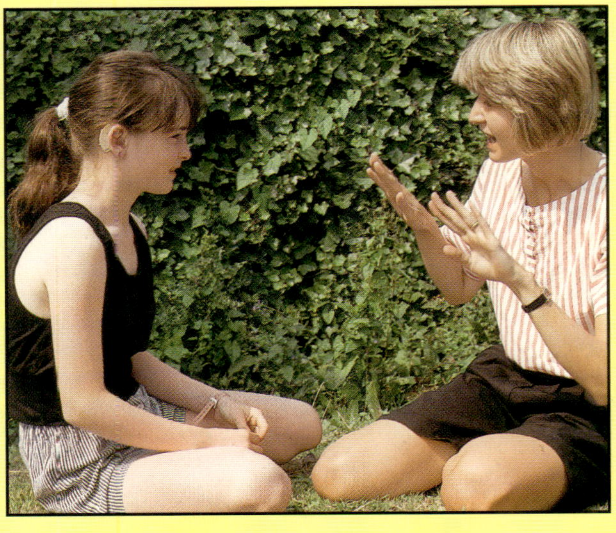

### Conversation

To help a deaf person to lipread, you should make sure that he or she can see your face clearly all the time. Do not stand in shadow or with your back to a bright light. You should talk naturally but not too slowly and speak as clearly as possible. It is not helpful to shout because this distorts the mouth patterns and makes lipreading more difficult. While you are talking, do not eat or smoke and avoid putting your hand over your mouth. Try to appreciate how difficult lipreading is and be prepared to repeat words.

## Learning to speak

Like all children, deaf children are born with the ability to learn and develop language. But deaf children find it difficult to learn speech because they have to imitate sounds they can see rather than sounds they can hear. And it is very difficult to control the sounds you make if you cannot hear the sound of your own voice.

A machine that lights up to show the loudness of speech helps deaf people to "see" the sounds they make and learn how to control them. Feeling the throat while speaking can also be helpful. The vibrations made by sounds give clues to how loud they are and when they are changing.

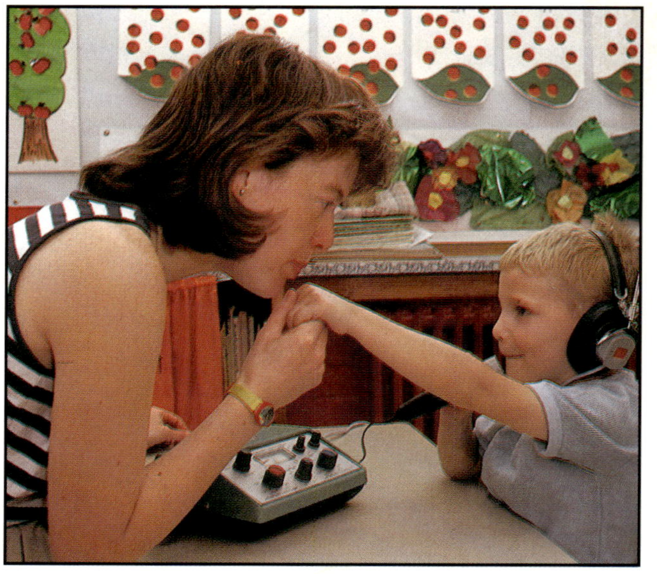

*Helping a deaf child become aware of sounds*

## Feeling the vibrations

If you hold a balloon near your mouth as you speak, you will feel the balloon vibrating. This happens because the balloon picks up the sound waves your voice makes. A balloon can be used to help a deaf child learn how to control the voice. The teacher speaks into the balloon and the deaf child feels the vibrations. The child then tries to make a sound which causes the same vibration.

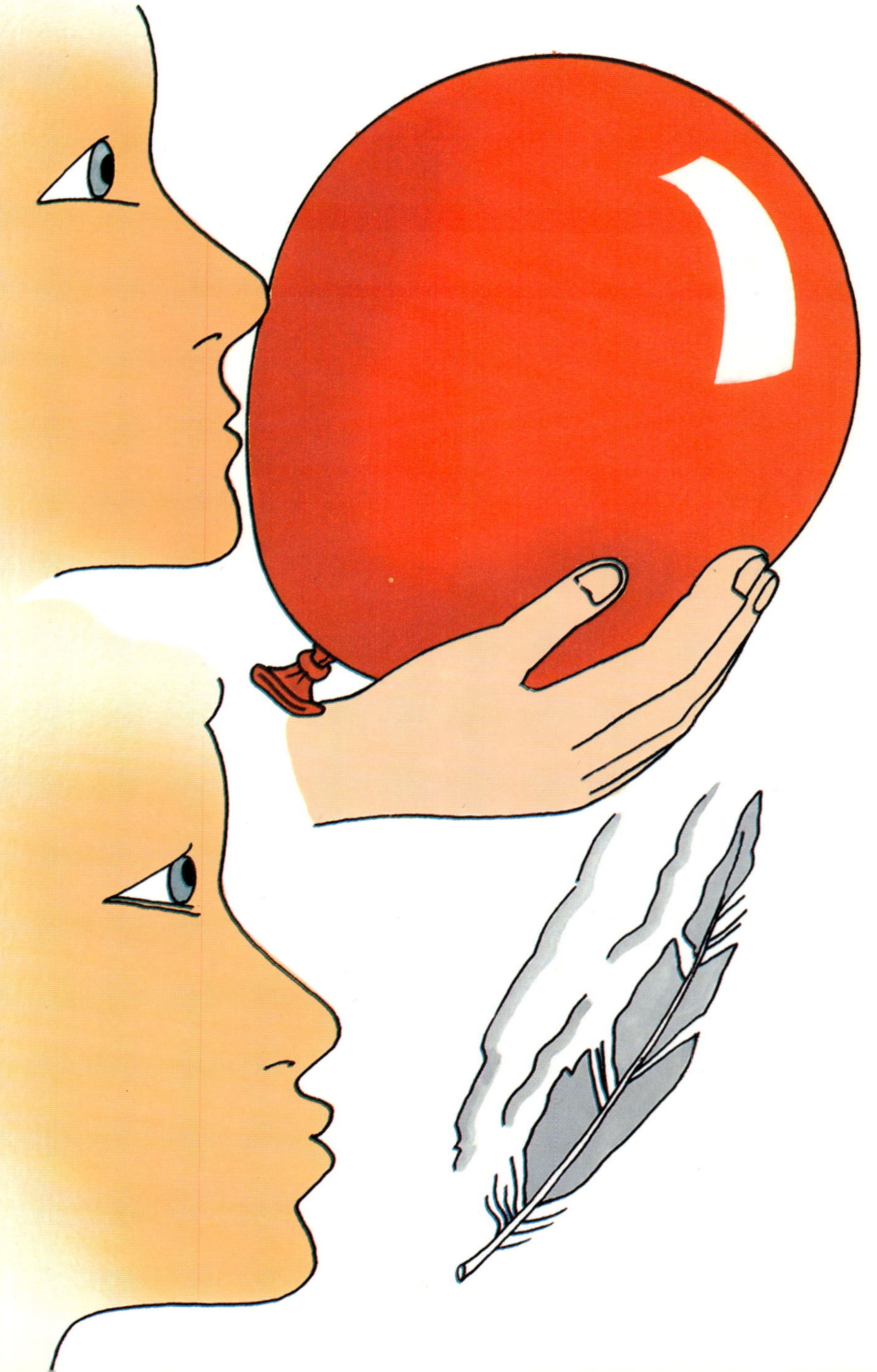

## Breath control

The noises we make when speaking are made by passing air over the vocal cords. The noises also depend on how we control the air with our lips and tongue. So to speak clearly it is very important to be able to control your breathing. Deaf people can practice a number of different exercises, such as blowing a feather, to try and improve their breathing and have control over it.

## Music

Children with a hearing loss have a range of interests and abilities. Depending on the level of their hearing loss, there is no reason why they should not enjoy music. Deaf people can feel sound vibrations and rhythms through musical instruments. Many learn to play musical instruments. Some partially deaf children are able to hear more high pitched notes well. As the ear is also the organ of balance, some kinds of deafness may affect a person's sense of balance and some people, particularly young children, tend to be more accident prone because of this.

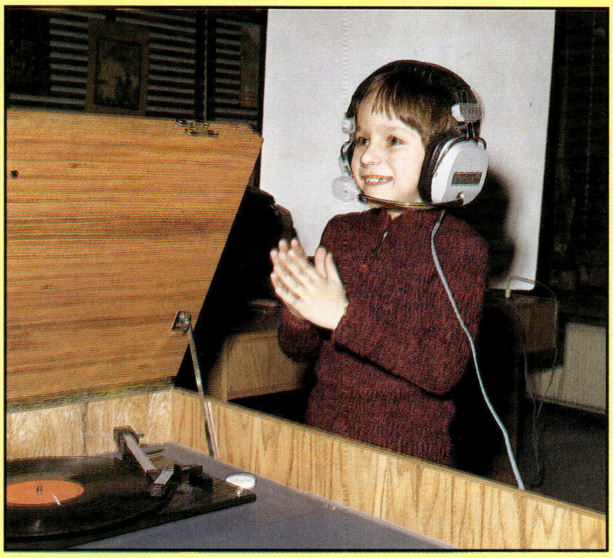

*Feeling rhythm through music*

## Losing the sense of sound

The brain begins to amass a store of sound memories from the moment of birth, and by adulthood people are able to distinguish nearly half a million signals that are meaningful. Should the sound memory center be accidentally destroyed, a condition called auditory amnesia occurs. Although nerve impulses corresponding to sounds do reach the brain, they no longer have any meaning. This is a difficult condition to treat because it is the brain, rather than the ear itself, that is damaged.

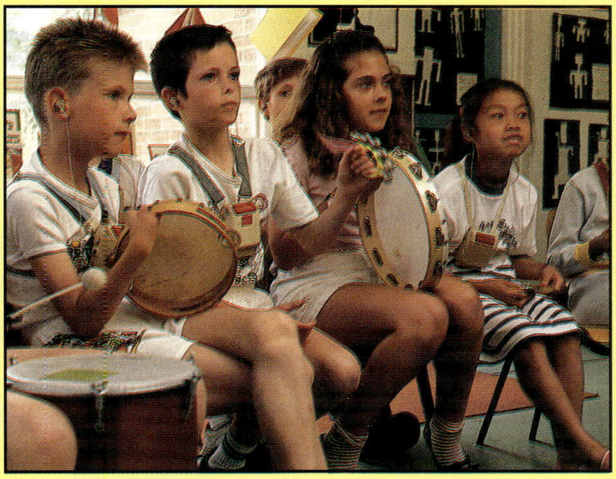

*Feeling sound through percussion instruments*

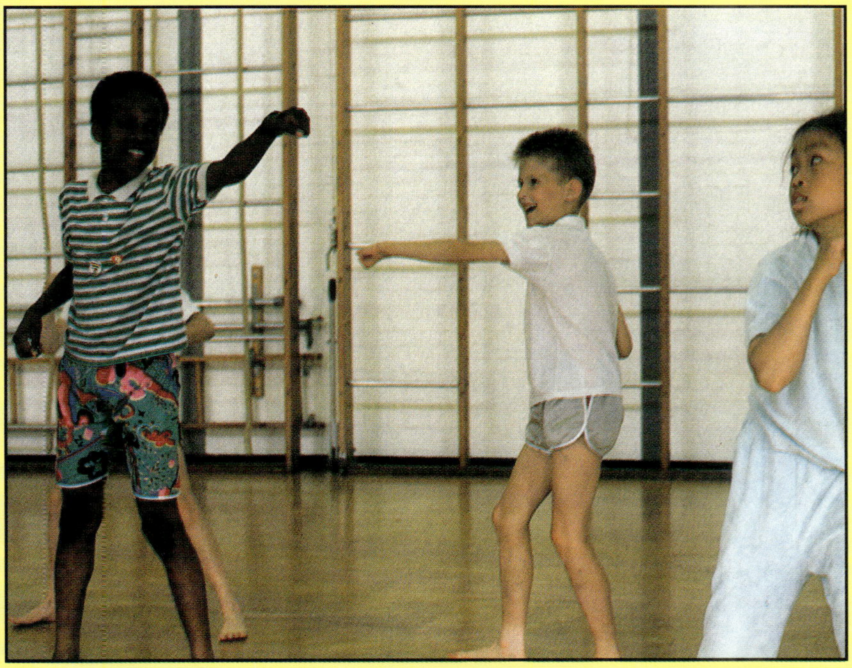

*Dance therapy helps coordination and balance*

## Dance

Deaf children can appreciate natural rhythms, even if they are profoundly deaf. So they may enjoy dancing and this can also help them to learn how to coordinate their movements. A loop system (see page 21) can help partially deaf children in this activity. It allows hearing aids to be used like a radio receiver. Music can be wired so that it is picked up by the children's hearing aid.

## LIVING WITH DEAFNESS

Children with a hearing loss are educated in ordinary schools as far as possible. Generally, the choice regarding the kind of education that a child with a hearing loss has is made according to parental preference – in the same way as any child's education. There are special schools available for children with hearing disabilities. In special schools the education is as wide as in ordinary schools but it is delivered by teachers who have had some training in the use of hearing aids and other equipment, as well as the use of sign language. Alternatively, some special schools maximize on the residual hearing of the pupils and use hearing aids without any signing systems.

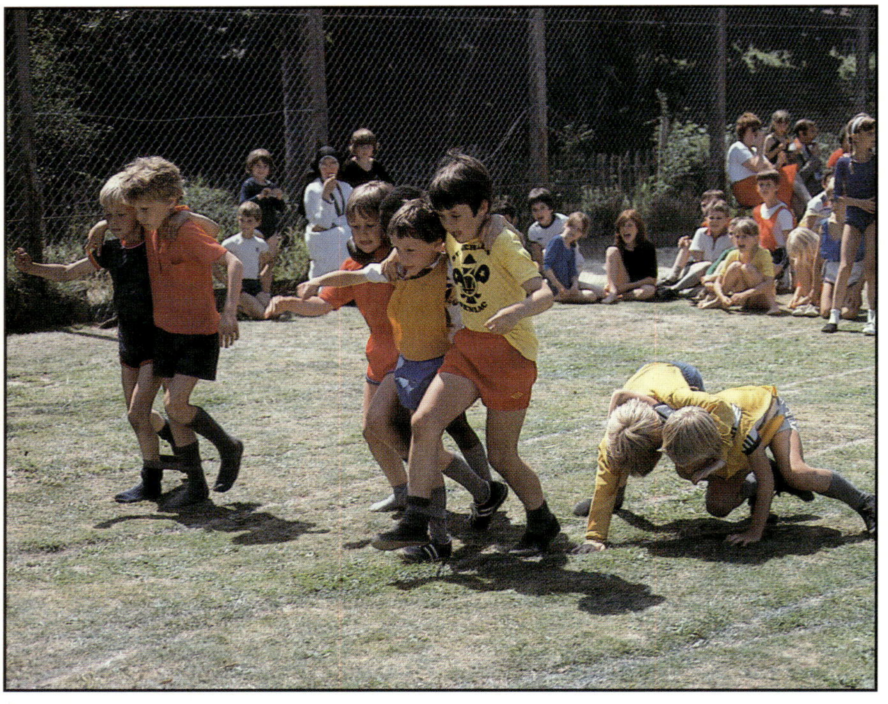

*Sports day is exciting for all children*

### At school

In some special schools for deaf children the teaching methods incorporate all kinds of communication – signing systems and hearing aids. Using "total communication" methods, deaf children are free to choose the best way of expressing their ideas and feelings. Deaf children have to work harder than hearing children in order to keep up with their lessons and so they are under more stress. Teachers should make allowances for this, and we all should be aware of emotional and social difficulties.

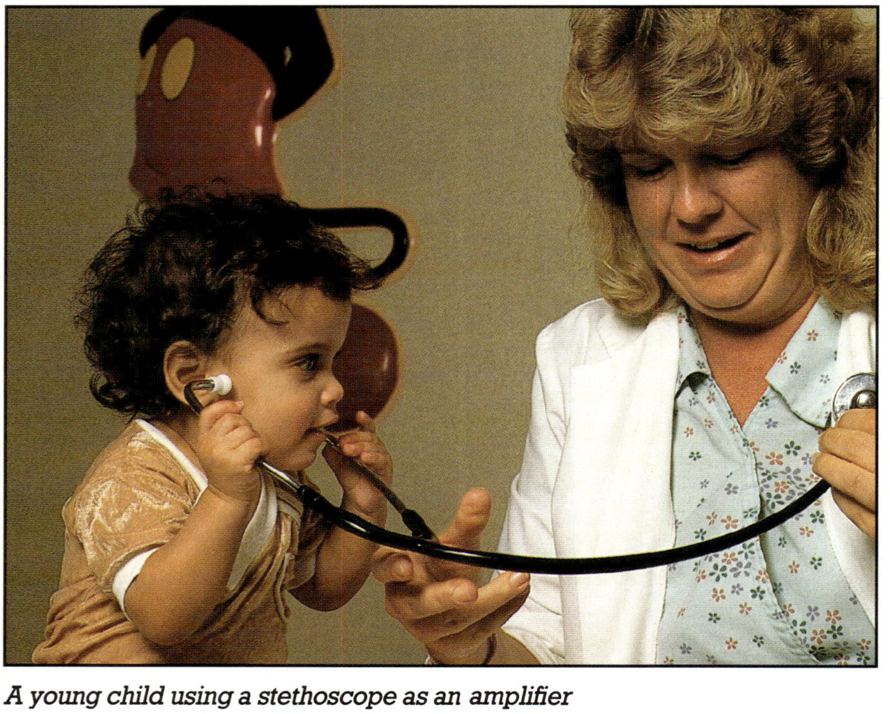

*A young child using a stethoscope as an amplifier*

### At work

There are many occasions when deaf people find an interpreter useful. These include telephone calls, job interviews, medical or dental examinations and conferences

### At home

The early formative years are vital for a child who is born deaf or has hearing problems. The family should try and help the child feel safe and comfortable so he or she is able to relax in a world without sound.

# LEADING A NORMAL LIFE

Approximately one child in every thousand is born profoundly deaf and mild or partial hearing loss is not unusual. It is important for everyone to understand that deaf children are certainly not dumb but they simply have difficulty in learning to speak. This is because they cannot hear other people's voices or their own – which is why their voices often sound strange. The more aware that people are towards the particular difficulties that deaf people encounter, the easier it is to adjust to the problems. In adults, the deafness caused by a gradual hearing loss in old age simply increases feelings of loneliness and isolation. Although deafness is a handicap, it is possible, particularly with help and care from others, for deaf people to lead a normal life. For young babies who are born with deafness, the world may seem to be a hard and frightening place to understand at first. But if a baby is stimulated during the first few formative years of life, he or she will probably grow up to be as well-adjusted and have the same kind of opportunities as other children who are not deaf.

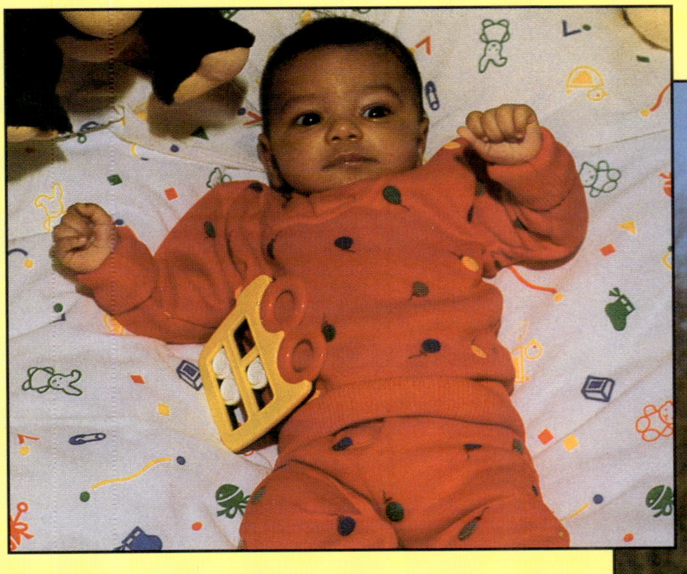

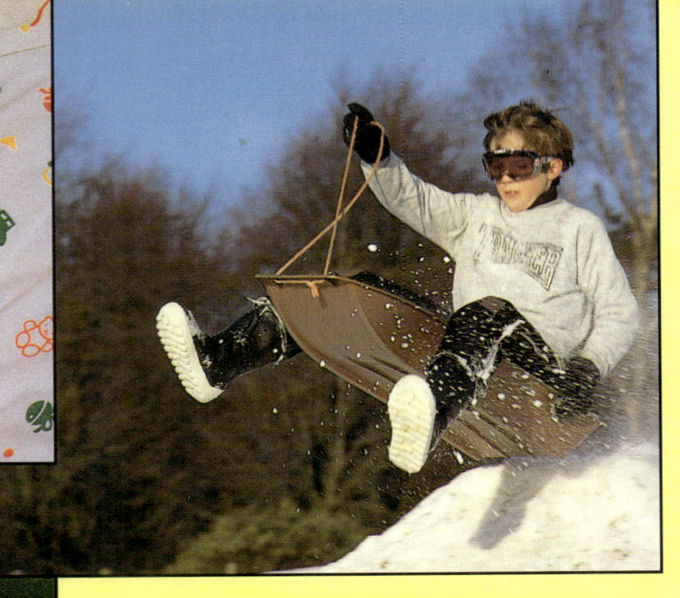

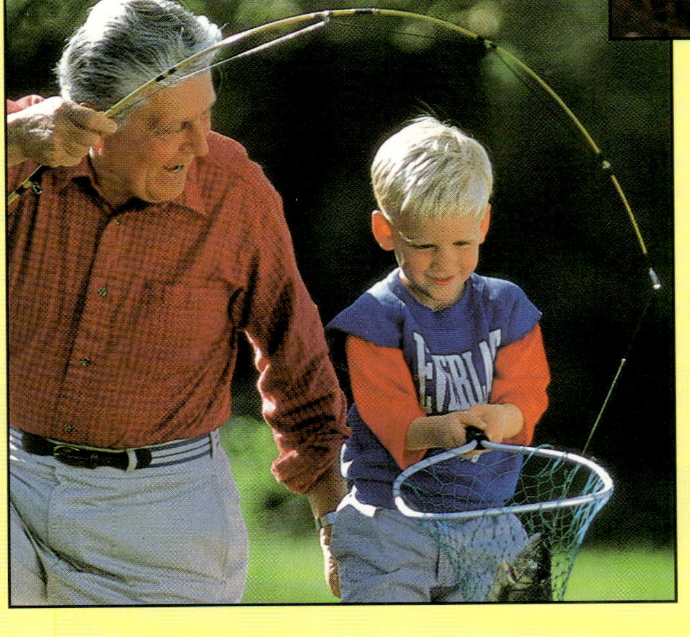

## Helping to communicate

When you speak to someone who is using a hearing aid, consider the problems they might have. It is important to reduce outside noise by shutting doors and windows. Face the person, keep your hands from your face and speak directly, because your listener may also be lipreading. It is important to speak slowly and distinctly – do not shout as this overloads the amplifier and distorts sound. Also try to avoid unnecessary background noises such as jangling keys and money.

# CARING FOR YOUR EARS

Many sounds can damage your hearing, including noisy aircraft, industrial machines and very loud music. If you are exposed to loud noise for a short while, you may feel slightly deaf for a time. But your hearing should slowly return to normal when you are out of the noisy environment. Too much loud noise, however, can lead to a permanent hearing loss.

A person firing a gun or using a chain saw should wear ear muffs to protect the ears. It is also a good idea to protect your ears if you use a noisy electric drill in a small space or for a long time. People in noise-producing occupations such as a road drill operator are at risk if they do not protect their ears from constant noise.

People often do not like to wear ear muffs or ear plugs because it cuts them off from other people and things around them. Some people's ears are more at risk than others, but it is impossible to find this out until damage has already occurred.

### Decibels

The loudness of sound is measured in units called decibels, or dB for short. Sixty dB is the loudness of conversation, and 120 dB that of a jet engine. If a person "loses" 25 dB of loudness, he or she may have a hearing difficulty. A loss of 95 dB can make a person almost totally deaf.

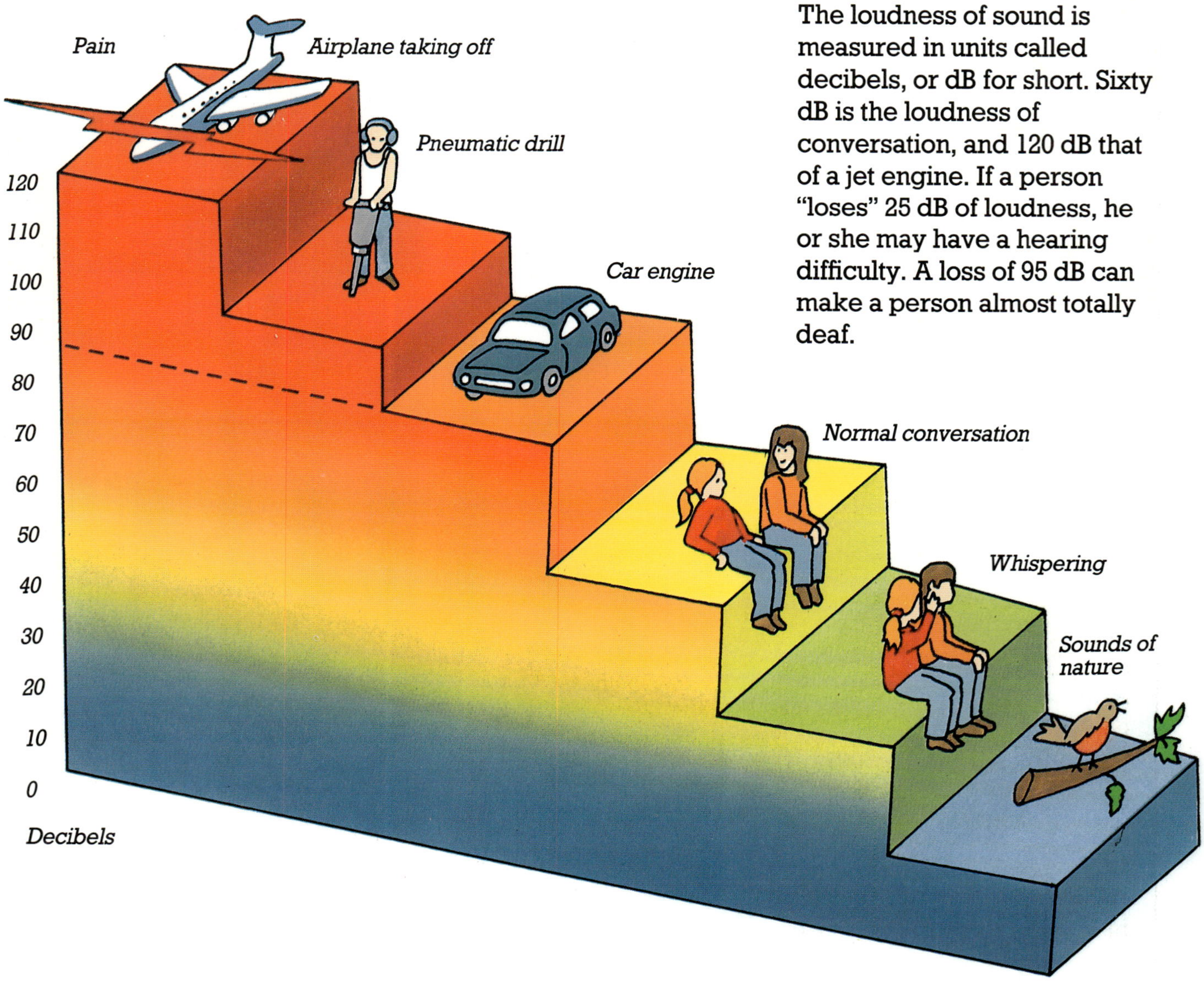

## Noise at work

Working in very noisy factories and industries impairs many people's hearing. The loud noise damages the sensitive cochlea in the inner ear. It is not just the amount of noise that is important, but also the length of time you are close to it. Laws have been passed to set the level above which a noise becomes dangerous. In the United States, the level is 85dB. If the noise is above this limit, employers should provide ear plugs or ear muffs. Safety officers check that ear protection is available and is being used in the correct way.

## Loud music

Constant bombardment of the ears with loud music at discotheques and pop concerts can also cause loss of hearing. Even the quieter modern bands can produce sound levels that are dangerously high. The noise level in an average discotheque can be as high as 120 dB – the same as from a jet aircraft. The people most likely to suffer are those running the shows because they have to listen to the loud noise night after night. Playing music too loudly on a personal stereo for long periods of time can also damage a person's hearing. This kind of problem can easily be avoided.

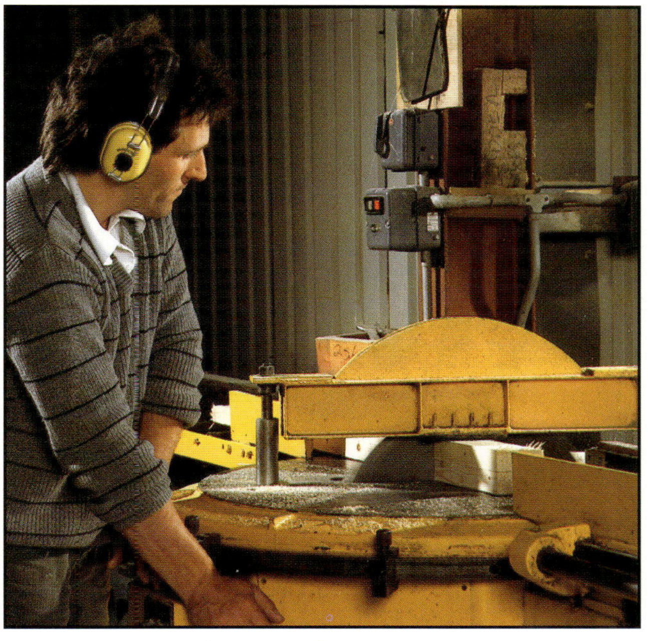

*Wear ear protection at work*

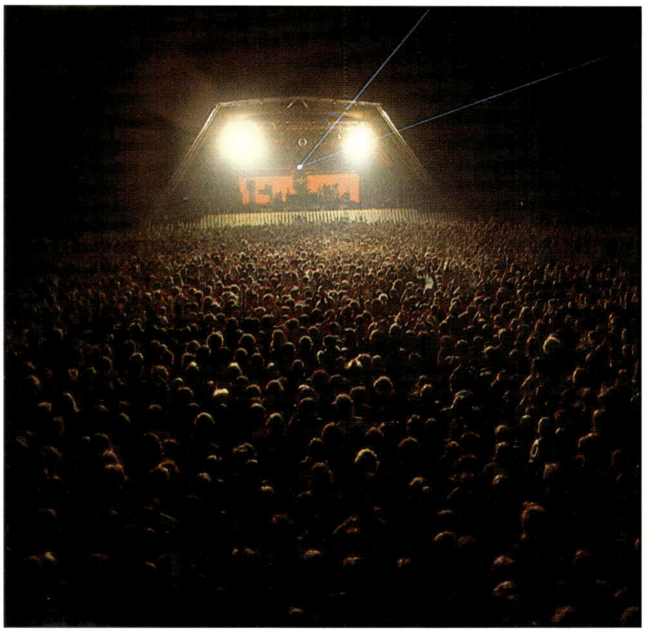

*Avoid standing near the speakers at concerts*

## In the water

If a person has a perforated eardrum or grommets (see page 15) in the eardrum, he or she should try to avoid getting water in their ears. If the water reaches the middle ear, it could cause infections or damage the ear. Wearing a bathing cap helps to prevent water entering inside the ears, especially if the person keeps the head above water. There is a silicon putty that a person can squeeze into their ear which creates a watertight seal. Used with a swimming cap it provides good protection against ear infections.

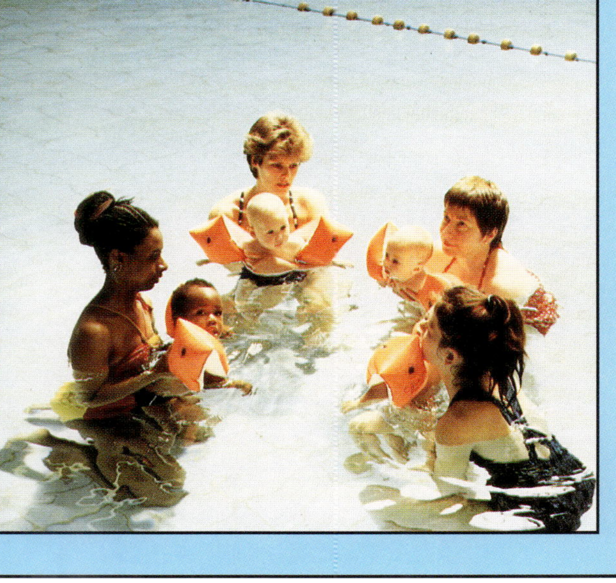

## FIRST AID

You should never push or poke anything into your ears to try and clean the ear canal. This can compress the ear wax into a hard lump and stop it moving out of the ear as it should naturally. The job of ear wax is to trap dirt and debris and carry it out of the ear. So if you leave your ears alone, they will clean themselves. There is also a risk that poking things into the ear may damage the eardrum and cause serious hearing problems.

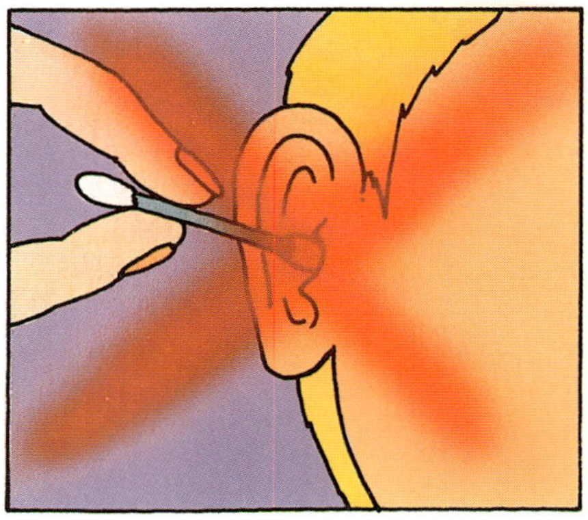

CLEANING
There is usually no need to clean your ears. The hairs and wax in the ear canal will do the job for you.

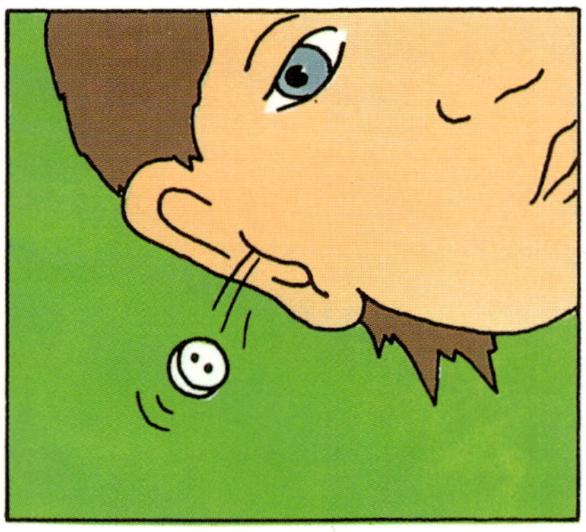

FOREIGN BODIES
If an object does become stuck in the ear canal, tilt the head to let it fall out and go to a doctor for help.

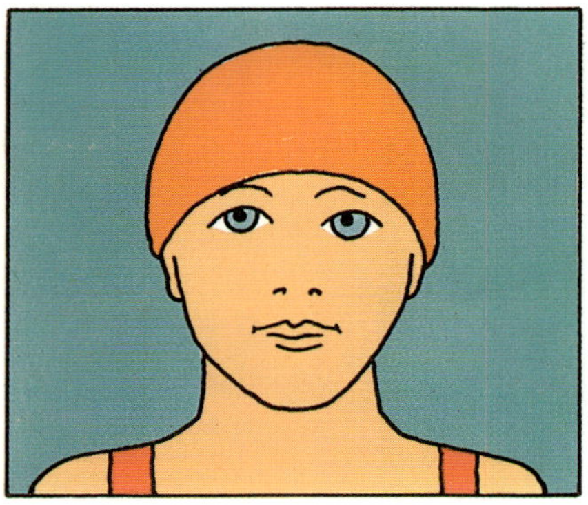

SWIMMING
If you have any ear problems, wear a cap when you go swimming.

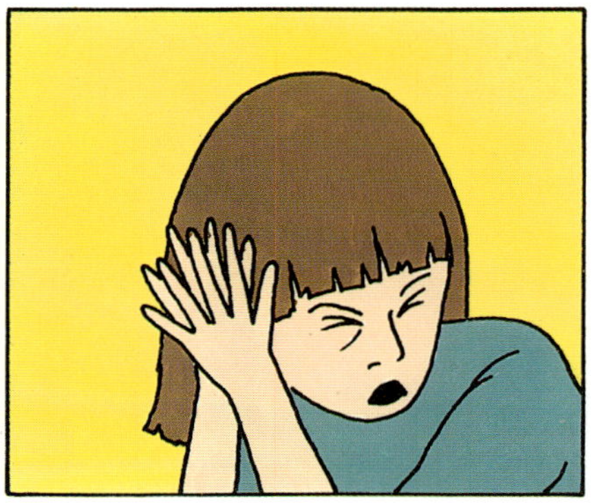

EARACHE
If you have an earache, you should go to a doctor for treatment as soon as possible.

Earaches are a sign that something is wrong with the ear. They can be caused by infections in the middle ear. This can lead to more serious disorders because the infection can spread to other parts of the body. Therefore, the sooner treatment can begin, the safer it is for you and the rest of the family. If you have any problems with your ears, go to a doctor for a check-up as soon as you can.

### Help and Information

National Association of the Deaf
814 Thayer Avenue
Silver Spring, MD 20910

Information and lists of materials relating to needs of deaf in education, research, rehabilitation, and employment.

American Speech and Hearing Association
10801 Rockville Pike
Rockville, MD 20852

Professional group providing services in speech and hearing; certifies professionals in field, etc.

Canadian Association of Deaf
56A Wellesley Street, E.
Toronto 284
Ontario, Canada

## GLOSSARY

**Audiogram** A chart showing the amount of hearing loss in decibels.

**Auditory nerve** The nerve that carries electrical signals (nerve impulses) from the cochlea to the brain.

**Cochlea** A bony structure in the inner ear which converts the frequency and loudness of sound into electrical signals.

**Cochlear implants** Tiny hearing aids which are implanted onto or inside the cochlea.

**Conductive deafness** A hearing impairment which affects the outer or middle ear. It can often be treated.

**Decibel** A unit used to measure the loudness of sound.

**Earmold** A piece of plastic, moulded to fit the shape of the ear, which conducts sound from a hearing aid into the ear.

**Eustachian tube** A tube leading from the middle ear to the throat.

**Fingerspelling** Using hand and finger shapes to stand for the letters of the alphabet.

**Frequency (pitch)** Sound vibrations per second, measured in hertz (Hz).

**Glue ear** A build-up of thick, sticky fluid in the middle ear, due to a blocked Eustachian tube.

**Grommet** A small plastic tube used to hold open a slit in the eardrum.

**Hearing aid** A device which makes sounds louder. It may be worn behind the ear (post-aural aid), on spectacles, on the body (body-worn aid) or in the ear.

**Lipreading** Trying to understand speech by "reading" the shape of the lips. In the United States, it is often called "speech reading".

**Loop system** A wire loop connected to the source of a sound. It gives out a magnetic field which a hearing aid converts back into sound again.

**Myringoplasty** An operation to repair a hole in the eardrum.

**Nerve deafness** This condition is also sometimes referred to as sensori-neural deafness. It is a hearing impairment which affects the inner ear or pathways to the brain. It causes distortion of speech and makes speech hard to understand. It cannot usually be treated medically.

**Otosclerosis** A condition in which the middle ear bones become covered with a bony growth and cannot vibrate freely.

**Oval window** The entrance to the inner ear. The interface between the ossicles and fluid-filled cochlea in the inner ear.

**Pure tone audiometry** A way of testing how well a person can hear a range of tones of one frequency only.

**Radio aid** A device which sends radio waves from one person to another. A radio receiver or a hearing aid converts the radio waves into sound waves and makes them louder.

**Sign language** A system of signs made with the hands. The signs stand for words or ideas.

**Total communication** A way of teaching that uses all forms of communication, including sign language, fingerspelling, speech reading, lipreading, drawing and writing.

# INDEX




**Photographic Credits:**
Cover and page 29b: Anthea Sieveking/Network; pages 5, 22 and 23: Roger Vlitos: pages 6, 10, 11 all, 16, 21, 29t and 29m: Science Photo Library; page 7: Magnum Photos; pages 8, 14 and 15 both: National Medical Slide Bank; pages 10 and 14: Biophoto Associates; pages 12 both, 13 all, 17, 18 all, 19 both, 20, 23, 24 and 25m and 25b: Janine Weidel; page 25t: Zefa; page 26: J. Allan Cash Library; pages 26 and 27t: Robert Harding; pages 27m and 27b: Images/Biophot Associates.




PRINTED IN BELGIUM BY proost INTERNATIONAL BOOK PRODUCTION

**How a Psychologist Manages His Investments**

Ira Pendleton is a middle-aged family man who practices psychology in a western state. After a few years as a professor at a southern university, Ira moved to the West and set himself up in private practice. He specializes in the treatment of children with learning problems. Over the years, Ira's practice grew from a one man operation to an incorporated clinic with seven other professionals. Although he will not be ready to retire for a number of years, Ira has begun to consider the type of support he will need during retirement. His retirement income will come from several sources: social security, income from the sale of his share of the clinic, a regular investment portfolio of stocks, and an Individual Retirement Account he manages himself. Ira has made a serious hobby of following a few selected stocks and the performance of several money market funds.

With substantial investments in several funds, Ira used a SuperCalc spreadsheet to make decisions about shifting his money between funds that invested only in bonds that produce tax-free interest income and funds with higher, but taxed, income. His spreadsheet allows him to enter the percent of payout for each fund, taxes which will be generated by income, and the actual after-tax gain for a person in his tax bracket. In addition, Ira uses SuperCalc to pose *what if* questions. What if rates go down on investments in taxable money market funds? What if interest rates rise, but personal income taxes go down?

Ira also uses SuperCalc to keep track of his total retirement income picture. Using estimates of likely performance of his different retirement income sources over the coming years, he has some idea of what he will have available if he retires at age 60, 62, 65, or later. For example, he found last year that a sustained downturn in interest rates over any two year period before 1988 would mean his retirement income would be less than his target amount. To compensate for that, he invested more in his IRA this year and plans to do the same again next year. If interest rates remain high, Ira will reduce the amount of income he puts into retirement related investments and use that money for something else. SuperCalc gives him more control over, and more involvement in, the way he spends his money.

Are the examples described above typical? Probably not. People regularly report applications of SuperCalc the developers never even thought about.

SuperCalc is a tool which can be used in many different ways. Essentially, it displays and manipulates information, particularly numeric information, and displays the relationships between different types of information. A bank loan officer may create a SuperCalc spreadsheet that displays mortgage payments for specific amounts spread across a variable number of years. It is very easy to enter new rates as interest rates change, and get accurate new tables. The tables may be printed out or simply displayed on the screen. An investment broker may keep track of real estate properties and estimate his income. A manager may use the program for cash-flow analysis and for her expense account. There may be as many uses as there are people who use it.

## A SHORT INTRODUCTION TO THE SPREADSHEET

A SuperCalc spreadsheet is arranged in columns and rows. There are 63 columns that are labeled across the top of the display with letters, from A to BK. The rows are numbered from 1 to 254 down the side of the display.

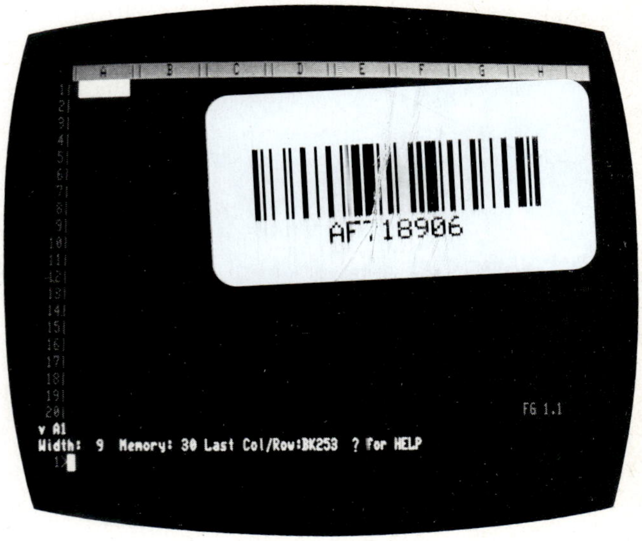


**Figure 1.1** The SuperCalc worksheet initially displays eight columns and twenty rows

Any point where a column or row intersects is called a *cell*. Cells are named by the row and column intersection. A cell found by coming down column D and across row 12 is called D12. SuperCalc thus operates on an electronic spreadsheet or worksheet that is 63 columns wide and 254 rows long. That means there are up to 16,002 individual cells into which information can be placed by you or by SuperCalc as it follows your directions.

You may now be wondering how a small video screen can display 16,002 cells on the screen. Does SuperCalc come with a powerful magnifying glass? Actually, even if a magnifying glass were provided, none of the currently available microcomputer systems is capable of creating that sort of display.

SuperCalc has another solution. It displays only a portion of the spreadsheet. In the standard arrangement, it will show a *window* that is 20 rows long by 8 columns wide. Initially, you see columns A through H and rows 1 through 20. Using SuperCalc commands or special keys on the computer keyboard, it is possible to view any portion of the sheet you wish. The *window* can be moved around on the spreadsheet so you see the cells of most interest to you. It is even possible to break up the sheet into different sections and display rows and/or columns side by side that are not normally adjacent.

SuperCalc has many powerful instructions that electronically duplicate the laborious "cut and paste" methods that have traditionally been used to create and manipulate worksheets.

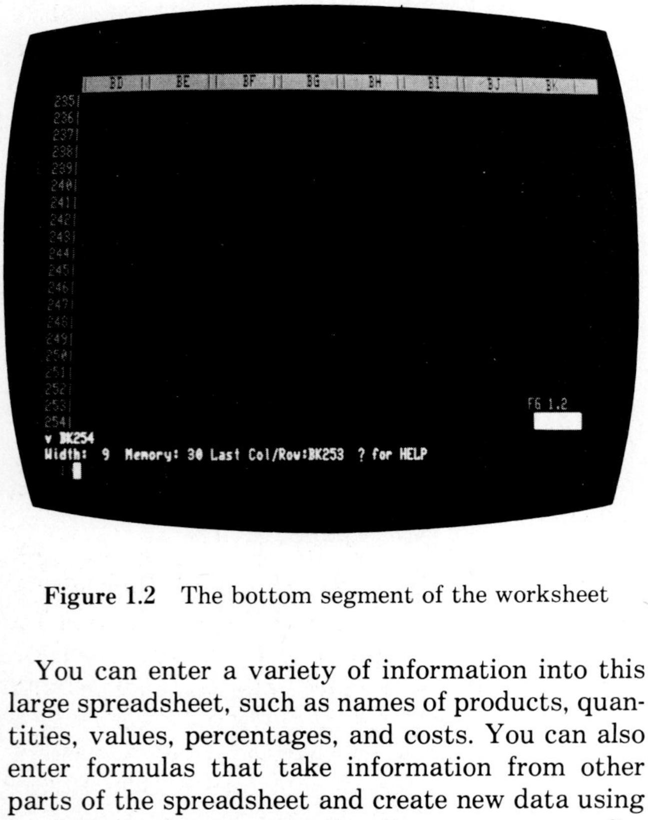


**Figure 1.2** The bottom segment of the worksheet

You can enter a variety of information into this large spreadsheet, such as names of products, quantities, values, percentages, and costs. You can also enter formulas that take information from other parts of the spreadsheet and create new data using math formulas you specify. Sums, averages, discount points, late payment penalties, and cost of service are a few of the many different types of calculations SuperCalc can perform for you.

This ability to organize, arrange, and manipulate data allows you to answer four different types of questions:

What happened?
What is happening?
What will happen?
What can happen?

By keeping track of past performance, SuperCalc can tell you exactly what happened in the past. For example, a firm which owns several rental properties can use SuperCalc to keep track of the performance of each piece of property. It can also tell you the current status of projects (what is happening), and can be used to generate a scenario of the future (what will happen). For instance, what will happen if the firm keeps a particular piece of property, and past trends in income, costs and tax/depreciation patterns continue? Finally, SuperCalc will answer *what if* or *what can happen* questions by allowing you to enter data reflecting a variety of decisions you *might* make in the future.

In today's quickly changing business environment, answers to any one of the four questions above can make the difference between success and failure. Even personal financial matters are often sufficiently complex to make SuperCalc an important personal tool.

Since SuperCalc is essentially a blank slate on which you create your own unique spreadsheet, its use requires some learning and practice. You will need to learn the rudiments of using a desktop computer. That will generally take no more than a few hours. Then you will need to learn a little about a program called CP/M (or a similar program that does the same job). Since SuperCalc is designed to operate in a computer which supports CP/M, we will deal with CP/M later in this section of the book. Finally, you will need to become familiar with SuperCalc itself. While you will be able to use some features of SuperCalc immediately, we estimate the minimum time required to really master SuperCalc is around 50 hours, spread, preferably, across several weeks or a month or two. For that investment of your time, you gain access to a powerful tool which can be customized to your special applications. Many people find they save far more than 50 hours of their time each year by using SuperCalc.

To help with the learning that lies ahead, two more introductory chapters will be presented in this section. The following chapter is an overview of small computers, and the next deals with the software used on them (including CP/M). The "preliminaries," the things you need to do to get SuperCalc up and running on your own computer, are covered in the Appendix. Generally, these preliminary tasks need to be performed only once. After that you can concentrate on learning to use SuperCalc.

This book is divided into three sections: the overview and introduction you are reading now, a tutorial section designed to teach you how to use SuperCalc, and a reference manual that provides succinct explanations and examples of all the instructions you can use in SuperCalc. The Tutorial Section is designed for the person who has training and experience in the intended area of application (e.g., banking and finance, or labor relations to name two) but who lacks extensive experience with computers. Most of SuperCalc's commands are covered in the tutorial.

SuperCalc is a well-designed program (one of the best we've seen), but, like most powerful tools, it is not simple. It has the power to meet sophisticated needs. If you are a first-time user we urge you to take the time to work through the Tutorial Section carefully. Take notes when you need to and complete the practice exercises.

After reading just the first chapters of the Tutorial Section, it is possible to begin using SuperCalc on your own (with occasional help from the Reference Section). You would not understand some of the finer points of the more sophisticated instructions, but you would be able to do many things with SuperCalc. There is, in fact, something to be said for learning the basics of SuperCalc first and then, after a month or two of experience, tackling the rest of the instructions.

Learning a piece of computer software such as SuperCalc involves more than memorizing the instructions. There is a certain rhythm to each piece of software, and there is a need to grasp and understand the inter-relationships between different functions and different instructions. This familiarity generally cannot be gained by working quickly through each individual instruction. It comes from working intimately with the program on a real or simulated task. In addition, some of the more complicated options in SuperCalc (explained in the Reference Section) are understood best by someone who is familiar with the operation of SuperCalc. It is then easier to see their usefulness and to understand where they are used most effectively. It is easy to "overrun" your level of mastery if you try to proceed directly through this book from cover to cover in a weekend. Be patient; spread learning sessions over several weeks, and you will find that SuperCalc is a very valuable tool in your profession or business.

## HOW TO GET THE MOST FROM THIS BOOK

Different people will use this book differently. You probably fall into one of the four following categories. Under each category, there are suggestions on how to get the most out of this book.

1. **Beginner who does not own SuperCalc.** Is SuperCalc something you can use in your business or profession? Is it difficult to use? To find out, read carefully Chapters 1 through 3 and the Appendix. Then read lightly Chapters 4 through 8. You should be able to get a feel for the program by reading these chapters and studying the screen displays. While you are doing this, you may want to look up some of the terms in the Reference Section.

2. **Beginner who owns SuperCalc.** If you would like to start doing something immediately, start with either the Appendix or Chapter 4. If you already know how to load the program, prepare diskettes for use, and so on, start with Chapter 4. Otherwise, start with the Appendix, and read Chapters 1 through 3 if you need an overview and introduction to computer software and spreadsheet programs. Then read carefully Chapters 4 through 8. Do it at the computer and work through the examples as they are presented. If you have a question about how a command or function works, look it up in the Reference Section. Then, once you have some experience using SuperCalc, read all of the Reference Section carefully. Initially, you will probably want to refer frequently to the Reference Section as you create your own worksheets.

3. **Experienced computer user who does not own SuperCalc.** If you are unfamiliar with electronic spreadsheets, you may want to begin by reading Chapter 1 (or finish it since you are near the end of Chapter 1 now). Then skim through Chapters 4 through 8. As with most good software, you can get a good feel for how a program works by reading the Reference Section.

If you are an experienced spreadsheet user considering a change to SuperCalc because of its superior features, you can probably become familiar with its features by reading the Reference Section.

4. **Experienced user who owns SuperCalc.** If you need help getting SuperCalc loaded and running on your computer, read the Appendix. Then, you might skim through the first chapters of the Tutorial Section to get a flavor of the program, but the Reference Section may give you all the information you need to use the program.

# Chapter 2

# The Basic Computer

This chapter will briefly describe the *hardware* that makes up a computer system. The term hardware refers to the nuts and bolts of a system, the physical equipment that you can see. However, hardware is only one half of a computer system. The other half is the *software*. The next chapter will cover software.

It is possible for you to purchase and use SuperCalc without knowing much about computer hardware. However, the "black box" approach does leave something to be desired. Some understanding of the components that make up a computer system, how they operate, and how they interface with each other can be very helpful. Such knowledge makes it less likely you will take something "on faith" and more likely you will understand why something is done in a certain way.

A typical small business computer is shown in Figure 2.1. The components inside the dotted lines are generally a part of the basic computer (memory, I/O, power supply, and CPU—these will all be explained in this chapter). The other components may be included in the basic computer or they may be *peripherals*. The term peripherals refers to equipment which is attached to the computer. Let's take a look at what each of the components in a small computer system does.

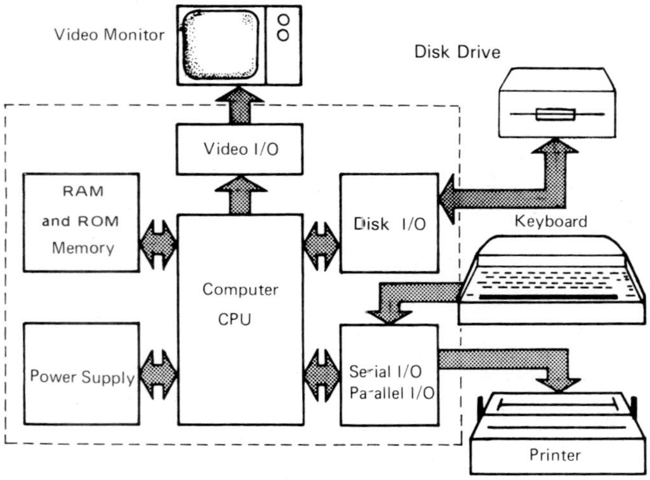


**Figure 2.1** A typical small business computer

## POWER SUPPLY

Most computer systems require at least two direct current voltages. The computer's power supply takes the 115 volts AC (alternating current) from your wall plug and converts it into the DC (direct current) voltages required by the computer.

The power supply also does another job. It filters the line voltage so that a circuit requiring +5 volts gets just that, no more and no less. Although most small computers require remarkably little power to operate, they are rather particular about their power. A large number of the problems associated with the use of small computers in homes and businesses are due to line voltage fluctuations. Significant drops in line voltage (e.g., "brownouts") may cause a computer to perform erratically. A number of companies sell special transformers that help your computer's power supply maintain a constant voltage to the system. Though expensive, they may be the only way to obtain dependable operation from a computer in environments with severe line regulation problems.

A related problem that can drive a computer user up the wall is the power line *glitch*. A glitch is a very brief spike of high voltage, often produced when a large motor is switched on or off (e.g., as in an air conditioner). The glitch may put several thousand volts on the power line for a split second; computers find it very difficult to digest glitches. Again, several companies manufacture devices which help keep glitches out of your computer.

## KEYBOARD

You "talk" to a computer through the keyboard. It is an *input device*. That is, it allows you to input information, instructions, or data to the computer. Keyboards vary considerably from system to system, but most look a lot like a standard typewriter keyboard. Many also have a *numeric keypad* on the right which looks like the keypad on a 10-key adding machine. The keypad makes it easy to input large amounts of numerical data into the computer.

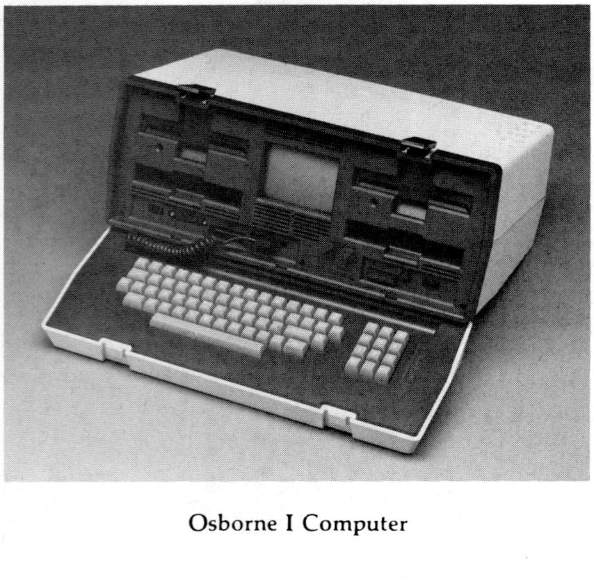

Osborne I Computer

Computer keyboards usually have a number of *function* keys. When pressed, function keys cause a particular action in the computer. For example, one key may tell the computer to clear the video screen of any information currently displayed. Another may tell the computer to send the information displayed on its video screen to the printer so that a permanent copy can be made. Function keys are handy and convenient since they allow you to tell the computer to do something by pressing one key. Keyboards without function keys often require you to press several keys in succession (or at the same time) in order to give the computer some instructions.

Many computers build the keyboard into the basic computer, others put the keyboard on a cord which can be plugged into the computer, and still others do not even provide a keyboard. For systems without their own keyboard, you must buy a *terminal* which contains a keyboard and a video display. Terminals will be discussed in the section on video displays.

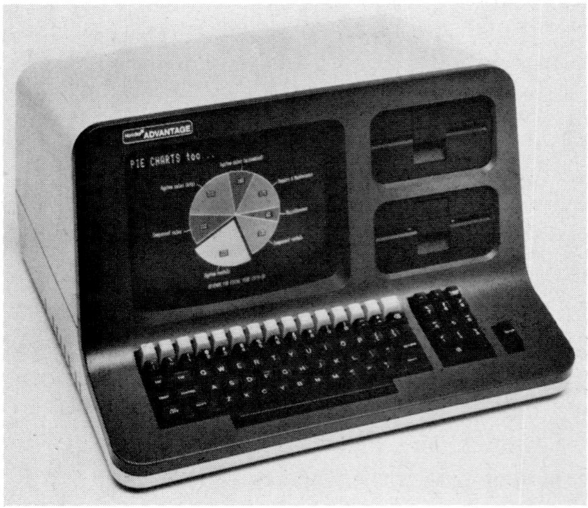


NorthStar Advantage

## VIDEO DISPLAYS

You talk to the computer through the keyboard. How does the computer talk to you? Most systems have two ways to *output* information to you: a printer and a video display. The video display looks a lot like a standard television; both use a CRT or cathode ray tube to display pictures or data. As you type in an instruction on the computer's keyboard, you will see what you typed on the video display. And, after you type in an instruction, the computer will generally respond by modifying or rearranging whatever is on the screen. You *input* on the keyboard; the computer *outputs* on the video display.

Video displays vary considerably in style, capacity, and options. Some display in black and white; others are a more eye-pleasing (and less fatiguing) green; and some can display in color. Many can display only standard upper and lower case letters, numbers and punctuations on the screen. The better displays can also show text material in several intensities. For example, you may see a frequently used business form on the screen with the printed material appearing in a light or half intensity print while the instructions on how to fill it out are in bold or double intensity print. The information you type in may appear on the screen in standard intensity. Then, when you finish filling in the form, the computer may take the information you typed in (the standard intensity text) and use it to fill out the form which is in the computer's printer.

Finally, displays vary in terms of capacity. Some are able to display no more than 12 lines of characters at once with 30 or 40 characters on each line. Most business computers can show 24 or 25 lines with up to 80 characters on each line. As with most things in life, the displays with more features generally cost more.

Most business computers use a *terminal* for video output and for input. A terminal is simply a device that contains a means to input data to a computer (usually a keyboard) and a means of displaying output from the computer (usually a CRT). You may hear the terms *dumb terminal* and *smart terminal.* A dumb terminal is generally only able to send and receive information from the computer. It cannot modify or edit the data being transmitted. A smart terminal may have enough "intelligence" to allow you to edit and change information on the terminal's screen before sending it to the computer. Some computers expect to be connected to a smart terminal and some can do nicely with a less expensive, dumb terminal.

## PRINTER

Video displays are popular because it is very easy to change and rearrange information on the CRT screen. For example, correcting typing errors in a letter is very easy on a display—not so easy on a typewriter. However, the image on a screen is not permanent. It disappears when the power is turned off. If you want a permanent *hardcopy* of the information on the screen, you must use a printer. Virtually all business computer systems, and many home computers, include at least one printer.

There are two major types of printer in common use today: dot matrix printers and letter quality printers. Dot matrix printers are less expensive; they usually print faster than letter quality printers. The quality of print produced by dot matrix printers is remarkably good considering their modest price. Dot matrix printers create the image of a character on the paper with a pattern of dots; the dots form the shape of the desired character. Letter quality printers are more expensive and generally slower, but their output is as good or better than that produced by an office typewriter.

## DISK STORAGE

If the printer provides you with a permanent copy, then the disk drive provides the computer with a permanent copy of material that may be used later. Programs, client records, research data, letters, reports and inventory records are all examples of material that is used over and over again by a computer. The computer cannot "read" or input information from the printed page, but it can "read" information stored magnetically on little platters of flexible material called *floppy diskettes.*

Floppy diskettes come in two sizes, 5¼-inch and 8-inch; they are used to store hundreds of thousands of characters of information. Most business computers use at least two disk drives to "read and write" information on diskettes. For example, as items are taken from a store's inventory, you can tell the computer what has been removed from inventory, via keyboard input. The computer takes the information and changes the magnetic codes on a diskette to reflect the current inventory status. If you need information on what is in inventory, the computer can read the information on the diskette and put the data on the video display or print it out on the printer.

Although floppy diskettes are the most common means of permanently storing information in a form the computer can use later, the *hard disk* is also gaining in popularity. It uses a solid metal disk for storage and is more expensive than floppy disk drives. However, hard disk systems can store millions of characters of data; they are very fast and they are very reliable.

## INPUT/OUTPUT CIRCUITS

Remember Figure 2.1? Thus far we have covered a way to input information and instructions into the computer (keyboard), ways the computer can output information to you (video display and printer), and a means of storing data in a format the computer can use (disk drives).

The figure also shows several I/O circuits inside the dotted lines that delineate the computer proper from the peripherals or accessories. I/O stands for *input/output.* An I/O circuit allows the computer to get input from external sources such as the keyboard and to output information to peripherals such as the printer and video display.

The I/O circuits in a computer generally get very little attention as long as they work properly. They do an important, but invisible, job. However, should you decide to buy a terminal, printer or special keyboard for your computer system, you will want to know what type of I/O your system uses.

Some computers offer both *serial* and *parallel* I/O circuits as standard equipment. Others consider either or both types of I/O as options that cost extra. Serial I/O circuits are required for virtually all terminals, many printers, and some keyboards. Parallel I/O circuits are required by many printers and keyboards and few, if any, terminals. The differences between serial and parallel I/O circuits will not be described here. There is more information about I/O circuits in *Computers for Everybody* by Jerry Willis and Merl Miller, and in *Peanut Butter and Jelly Guide to Computers* by Jerry Willis and Deborrah Smithy-Willis. Both are available from dilithium Press.

## MEMORY

A disk drive permits the computer to "warehouse" large amounts of information the computer may need later. However, material stored on a diskette is not immediately available for use. For example, suppose you have a SuperCalc spreadsheet for a particular application. Each time you use the spreadsheet you tell the computer to get it from the diskette where it is stored. The computer reads the data on the diskette and puts that data into *memory*. This process is like sending someone out to the warehouse to retrieve an item which is to be placed on the showroom floor, where it can be used.

A computer's memory works much like human memory. Information or data is stored as electrical charges in memory *cells*. These cells are actually tiny sections of silicon inside an integrated circuit or *chip* whose state can be changed by an electrical impulse. The computer can store electrical codes for letters, numbers and other characters in its memory, and then "read" each cell to determine what is stored there.

As shown in Figure 2.1, there are two major types of memory, ROM and RAM. ROM stands for *read only memory*. This kind of memory is programmed at the factory. It may contain instructions the computer will follow to perform a particular job. ROM cannot be changed by the user or by the computer.

The other type of memory, RAM or *random access memory*, can be programmed or changed as well as "read" by the computer. RAM is general purpose memory. You can store data or instructions in RAM, tell the computer to use the information you've stored there and then replace the material in RAM with something new. The biggest problem with RAM is that whatever is in it disappears when the computer is turned off. If you need to save something in RAM for use later, you must store it on a diskette before the computer is turned off (material in ROM remains there essentially forever).

## THE CPU

Finally we come to the heart of the computer system, the CPU or *central processing unit*. The CPU in a small computer is actually one relatively small integrated circuit or *chip*. Although most CPU chips are smaller than an Oreo cookie, the electronic components they contain would have filled a room a few decades ago. Using advanced microelectronic techniques, manufacturers can cram tens of thousands of circuits into tiny layered silicon chips that work dependably and use less power than an electric razor.

Several manufacturers make CPU chips today. Intel makes the 8080, 8086, and the 8088. Zilog makes the Z80 and Commodore makes the 6502. Though different in several ways, all the CPU chips do the actual processing inside the computer. The CPU also sends signals which synchronize the operation of each component in the computer system. This synchronization permits the system to perform thousands of operations a second. These operations are fairly simple (e.g., adding two numbers together) but the speed at which they are performed allows the computer to do some very complex things. The computer breaks down complicated jobs into hundreds of simple steps.

All the hardware that makes up your computer system is little more than a bunch of parts if there are no instructions that tell the computer what to do. Those instructions are the focus of the next chapter.

# Chapter 3

# Computer Software

If computer hardware seems mysterious, computer software must seem doubly so. If the computer were a kitchen (with the CPU the stove) the software would be a recipe. Just as there are many different types of recipes, so too are there many different types of software.

## LANGUAGES FOR COMPUTERS

The computer in your home or office probably speaks several languages. No, it won't converse fluently in French or Spanish, but it probably will speak BASIC, maybe Pascal, and probably some dialect of a cryptic group of languages called *machine language*.

The particular CPU chip used in a computer determines which machine language it speaks. For example, the NorthStar Advantage computer uses the Z80 CPU chip. Not surprisingly, it speaks Z80 machine language. The Commodore PET computers use the 6502 chip and speak 6502 machine language.

Although much commercial software (including SuperCalc) is written in machine language, most beginners will want to leave that language to the experienced programmer. Machine language is hard to use, and very tedious and time-consuming for the programmer. Learning it requires dedicated study. Machine languages also use strange number systems (hexadecimal, octal, binary) instead of the familiar favorite, decimal. Here is an excerpt from a machine language program:

```
04000 072   LDA A
04001 037
04002 004
04003 117   MOV C,A
```

All the numbers are written in octal, a base 8 number system. The first column of numbers (e.g., 004000) specifies the memory cell in the computer where the instructions are located. Computers don't understand words or letters, so everything must be converted to numbers before the CPU chip can determine which instruction it is supposed to carry out.

The 072 in the first line of this excerpt will cause the computer to perform a particular function. CPU chips are designed to execute any of several hundred different instructions, and each instruction has a number associated with it. When the CPU chip "reads" a memory cell and finds the number of an instruction there, it executes or performs the function associated with that number. Programming in machine language involves writing out a list of those instructions for the computer to follow and storing them in the memory of the computer.

The last column in the program excerpt lists a sort of shorthand summary of what the computer will do as the instructions are followed. For example, the term LDA means "load the accumulator with the contents of the memory location indicated by the number that follows." (The accumulator is a special memory location inside the CPU). MOV C,A means "move whatever is in storage location A to storage location C."

The computer deals only with the numbers in the second column, the machine language instructions. The first column indicates where the instruction will be placed in the computer's memory, and the third column is for humans who want to read the listing of a machine language program to figure out what is happening. A program called an *assembler* allows you to type in instructions like MOV C,A and have them automatically converted to machine language instructions.

It takes tens of thousands of machine language instructions to make up a sophisticated program like SuperCalc. Fortunately, you will not have to learn machine language to use SuperCalc. The programmers have done the hard work for you!

## HIGHER LEVEL LANGUAGES

This family of languages uses English-like words and mostly decimal numbers for programming. The best known of these languages is BASIC; it is fairly easy to learn. Here is an example of a BASIC program:

```
10 PRINT "HELLO, WHAT IS YOUR NAME?"
20 INPUT N$
30 PRINT "WELL ";N$;", I AM GLAD YOU
   CAME OVER TO TALK TO ME."
```

As you can see, BASIC is more familiar than machine or assembly language. In BASIC, each line of instructions for the computer has a line number. The three lines shown here are numbered in increments of 10. They could just as well be numbered in increments of 2, 20, or 3. The computer doesn't care. However, it will begin with the line with the lowest number, execute the instructions in it, and then proceed to the line with the next lowest number, and so on.

A computer that "speaks" BASIC understands a set of *keywords* which have a specific meaning for the computer. In the example, the keywords PRINT and INPUT were used. Another keyword in BASIC is RUN. If you typed the three-line program into your computer and then typed RUN, the computer would begin executing the program. That is, it would look at the line with the smallest number (in this case 10) and follow the instructions given there. Line 10 tells the computer to print the material between the quotations marks on the screen. Thus

**HELLO, WHAT IS YOUR NAME?**

would appear on the screen.

The keyword in line 20 is INPUT. That tells the computer to stop and wait for you to type in something on the keyboard. Suppose you type in CHARLIE. The computer takes CHARLIE and assigns it the label N$. Now N$ equals CHARLIE. In line 30, the computer finds another print instruction. It will print the following on the screen:

**WELL CHARLIE, I AM GLAD YOU CAME OVER TO TALK TO ME.**

The computer printed everything inside quotation marks just as it appeared (e.g., WELL, and I AM GLAD YOU CAME OVER TO TALK TO ME.). The N$ is not enclosed in quotation marks, however. Instead of printing N$, the computer looked at its list of labels and found that N$ stands for CHARLIE. Thus it printed CHARLIE on the screen instead of N$.

BASIC is, without question, the most popular small computer language today. More people work with BASIC than any other computer language, even FORTRAN and COBOL, two older languages which are used in scientific work (FORmula TRANslator) and in business (COmmon Business-Oriented Language). There are also at least a hundred other higher level languages, each with a group of supporters who believe their language is the best. Some of the other languages are specialized. For example, PILOT is designed primarily for educational applications. Others are general purpose languages which were developed because someone saw deficiencies in the currently available languages. One of these general purpose languages, Pascal, is finding a large following among small-computer users. Some say that in a few years it will replace BASIC as the most popular language for small computers.

## PROS AND CONS OF LANGUAGES

As noted earlier, computers themselves really speak only one language, machine language. You are able to write or use programs written in other languages such as BASIC only because the manufacturer of your computer developed a machine language program that takes your BASIC instructions and translates them into machine language instructions the computer can understand. The instructions that do the translating must be stored in the computer's memory (e.g., in ROM or in RAM) thus limiting the memory available for other uses. In addition, translating takes time. That means BASIC programs are generally quite a bit slower than programs written in machine language.

These two disadvantages, greater use of memory space and slower execution, are balanced against the ease of writing programs in higher level languages such as BASIC. Generally, it will take less time, and cost less, for a company to write a program it plans to sell commercially in a higher level language. If the program does not make large demands on the computer's memory space, and if speed of execution is not a problem, there are significant advantages to programming in higher level languages. However, some programs, including SuperCalc, do need all the memory available in the computer and they perform many complicated calculations and manipulations. Speed and memory conservation are thus important. In such cases, machine language programs offer a distinct advantage. Word processors are another type of program that are written almost exclusively in machine language since they use large amounts of memory and require fast execution.

## TYPES OF COMPUTER SOFTWARE

A difficult concept for many novices is the fact that there are different *types* of software that run in their computers. This section covers four types of software: languages, operating systems, utility software and applications software.

### Languages

Computer languages have already been discussed. Some computer manufacturers put the instructions that enable their system to "speak" BASIC, Pascal and other higher level languages in ROM (read only memory). If BASIC is in ROM, the computer is usually ready to speak BASIC when it is switched on. Other manufacturers put BASIC and other languages on diskettes. That means you must tell the computer to find the instructions on the diskette and put them in RAM (random access memory) before it can speak BASIC.

### Operating Systems

An operating system is a set of instructions, written in machine language, that lets you use all your computer components as an integrated computer system. For example, operating systems allow you to tell the computer to send information to the printer, the disk drive or the video display. The operating system software is usually in ROM and thus available for use as soon as the computer is switched on. Since most small business computers use diskettes for data storage, the operating systems that contain instructions for disk drive operation are called Disk Operating Systems or DOS. A common pattern today is to put just enough of an operating system in ROM to allow the computer to load a larger DOS into RAM from a diskette.

### Utility Programs

A utility program does work very similar to that of an operating system. A utility program is written to accomplish a specific, but routine, job. For example, there are several utility programs that enable you to use your small computer as a terminal to communicate with larger computers over the phone. Another type of utility program checks to see that your RAM and ROM, your disk system and your video display are all operating properly. Some diagnostic utility programs even tell you which chip needs to be replaced!

### Applications Software

Applications software is the type of software that you deal with most directly. An applications software package does something useful. Game programs, word processors, accounting software, and electronic spreadsheets are all examples of *applications software.* Applications software can be written in a higher level language like BASIC or in machine language. The distinguishing feature is that applications software is designed to solve a specific class of user-oriented problems. There are tens of thousands of applications programs available today for small computers. They range in price from less than $10 for a simple game program to well over $10,000 for a special purpose business program (e.g., a program designed for grain elevator operators or a program that keeps track of pharmacy prescription records).

### The Special Case of CP/M

One of the problems faced by companies that write applications software for small computers is the issue of operating system compatibility. For example, a program written to operate on a Radio Shack Model II computer must be set up to operate under Radio Shack DOS (disk operating system). Unfortunately, that DOS is not compatible with the DOS of other computers such as NorthStar, Apple, Cromemco and Vector Graphic. That means a software developer must write different programs for each brand of computer – a costly and time-consuming task. Fortunately, there is an alternative.

A company called Digital Research developed a disk operating system called CP/M, for Control Program for Microcomputers. It is not written for a particular computer. Instead, there are versions of CP/M for hundreds of different computers. CP/M is the closest thing to a "universal" disk operating system for small computers. If you own a computer that can use CP/M, you have a choice of buying applications software that runs under the version of DOS designed specifically for your computer, or software that runs under CP/M.

Since it takes thousands of hours to produce a major piece of applications software, many software companies prefer to write programs that run under CP/M. That way the same amount of effort produces a program that can be sold to owners of many different brands of computers. SuperCalc is one of many business applications programs that runs under CP/M. There are many different operating systems for computers today, and there are several that make an effort to be "universal" like CP/M. For the moment, however, CP/M is the most widely accepted operating system with a wider range of business software available than any other competitor.

To use SuperCalc in your computer, you must first load CP/M into memory from diskette. Then, after CP/M has taken control, you tell CP/M to load and run SuperCalc. The process of getting CP/M ready to run SuperCalc is the topic of the Appendix.

# TUTORIAL SECTION

## Chapter 4

# The Essentials of SuperCalc

The best way to learn how to use anything is through practice, and that's exactly what you'll do in this section. The purpose of this chapter is to introduce you to the basics of SuperCalc through a series of examples. Topics covered in this chapter include how to load SuperCalc, what a worksheet is, what its parts are and ways to put the program to work. The next chapter concentrates on specific examples of various instructions in SuperCalc. Chapters 6 and 7 also use specific examples, such as an expense account, to introduce the remaining major SuperCalc functions and commands. Throughout this tutorial section you will have opportunities to try various aspects of the program on your own. There will be examples for you to work out, and explanations of why things work as they do. So, if you're ready, here is SuperCalc!

### LOADING SUPERCALC

This is a brief explanation of how to load SuperCalc diskettes into your computer. If you're not sure how this is done, or if some of the terms are unfamiliar, you may want to read the Appendix for more detailed information. Formatting a diskette is also explained in the Appendix; you can follow the step-by-step instructions given there on how to format a diskette if you have not already done so.

If your computer is turned on, you are ready to begin. Switch the computer on and place the SuperCalc diskette (it should have both CP/M and SuperCalc on it) in your systems disk drive (this is either Drive A or Drive 0). Place a formatted disk in Drive B (assume that your second drive is called Drive B, even though on the system you have, it may be Drive 1 or something else). Remember to gently push the diskette into the drive until it *seats* or clicks in place, then close the door on the disk drive.

When your diskettes are in place, a red light on your disk drive will probably flash on. This light tells you that the computer is reading information from your diskette. Within a few seconds, your first communication with the computer will begin. Your screen should look similar to the one shown in Figure 4.1.

The first line tells you the manufacturer of your system. The second line lets you know that 64K of memory (see the Appendix for an explanation of memory) is required and that a particular version of CP/M is controlling the computer. In Figure 4.1, the CP/M version in use is 2.21, but yours may be a different version.

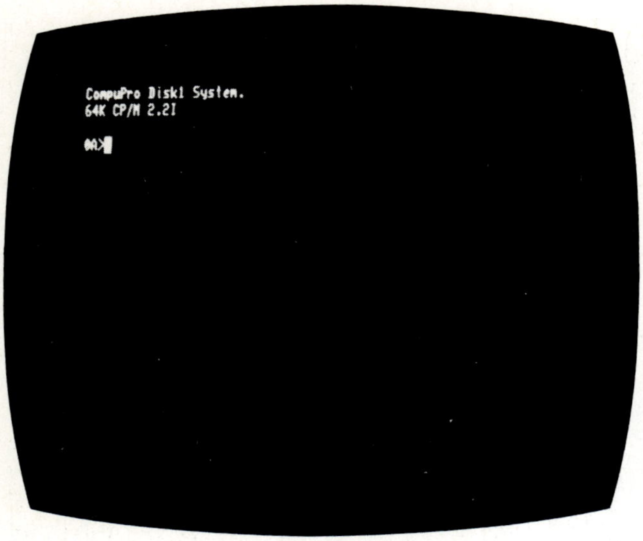


**Figure 4.1** The first screen you will always see

The **A>** is called a *prompt*. That is, the computer is letting you know that it is ready to follow your instructions. Different prompts are used throughout SuperCalc and each will be described later. Right now, the prompt **A>** lets you know the computer is waiting for your directions. In order to give directions, you must type the necessary instructions on the keyboard. The **A** means CP/M has designated Drive A as the primary or *system drive*. At this point you want to tell CP/M to find the SuperCalc program on the diskette in Drive A, load it into the computer's memory, and begin executing it. You might think the instructions to do all that would take one or two lines, but you don't even have to type in the entire name of the program. The abbreviation *SC* will do. In fact, typing the full name has no meaning at all to your computer. It also doesn't matter whether you use upper or lower case letters. Notice the white box at the end of the **A>**? That box is called the *cursor*. It tells you where the typed information will appear on the screen. On your computer or terminal, the cursor may be shown on the screen in a different way.

Remember we said that typing in the word SuperCalc would have no meaning to the computer? Try it and see. After the prompt **A>**, type

**SuperCalc**

and press the key marked **RETURN**. (From now on we will use the symbol [RET] to indicate that it is necessary to push the key marked **RETURN**. If you don't have a **RETURN** key, you probably have a key labeled **ENTER** instead.) The purpose of the **RETURN** key is to let the computer know you have finished typing a set of instructions and that it's time for the computer to execute those instructions. Thus, every time you see [RET], you should push the **ENTER** or **RETURN** key.

What happened when you typed in SuperCalc? Most likely your computer responded with the following message:

**SuperCalc?**
**A>**

It has no idea what SuperCalc or SUPERCALC or supercalc is. SuperCalc is stored on the diskette under the name SC. To get the program to work, all you have to do is type **SC**. Notice the **A>** prompt again. Now type

**SC**[RET]

When you typed **SC** after the prompt, you told the computer to read the SuperCalc program from your diskette into the computer's memory. The disk drive will run for a few seconds (the red light may come on again) and your first SuperCalc messages will appear. A screen similar to the one shown in Figure 4.2 will be displayed on the screen.

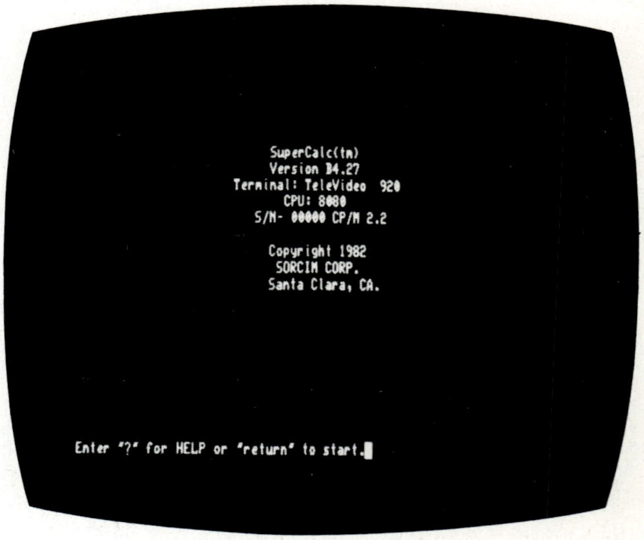
SuperCalc(tm)
Version B4.27
Terminal: TeleVideo 920
CPU: 8080
S/N- 00000 CP/M 2.2
Copyright 1982
SORCIM CORP.
Santa Clara, CA.
Enter "?" for HELP or "return" to start.

**Figure 4.2** The SuperCalc message screen

This screen provides you with some general information about the program. The first line tells you the name of the program, SuperCalc obviously. The second line lets you know which version of SuperCalc you have purchased. Next is information on which terminal or computer (i.e., Televideo, IBM, NorthStar, etc.) your version is set up to use. If this is not the system or terminal you have, you may have to check back with your dealer. Since SuperCalc is customized for each type of computer system, it is necessary to use the correct version of SuperCalc or risk unusual or inaccurate performance. (However, popular terminals such as the

ADM3 and the DEC series are often *emulated* by other manufacturers. Your terminal may be compatible with a version of SuperCalc that lists another brand on the screen.) The fourth line tells you what type of CPU (central processing unit) your version expects (i.e., 8080 or Z80). S/N is the serial number of your particular program. If you need help, and you call either Sorcim or your dealer, you may be asked for this number. The CP/M # refers to the version of CP/M your SuperCalc works with. Next is the copyright date, followed by the name Sorcim, the producers of SuperCalc, and where they are located.

Notice the message that is displayed across the bottom of the screen:

**Enter "?" for HELP or "return" to start**

This message lets you know that you can stop what you are doing at any time and ask for help. All you have to do is type the question mark ?; this will be explained later. The screen tells you to press RET to continue, so press RET and look at the blank SuperCalc worksheet. After pressing RET, your screen should look like the one shown in Figure 4.3.

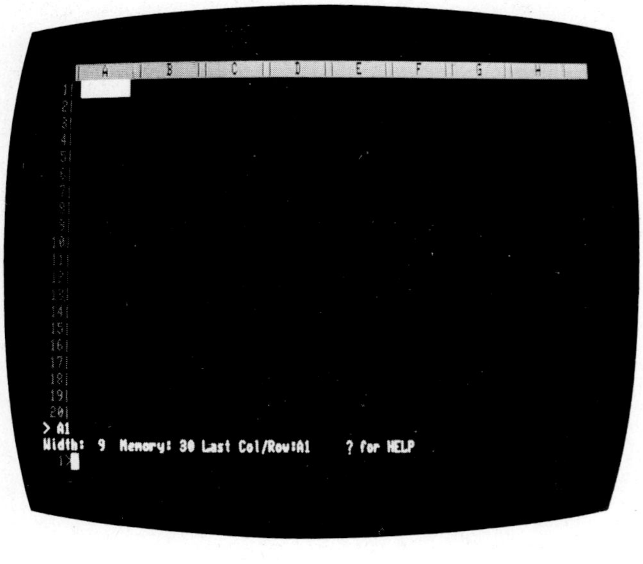


**Figure 4.3** A blank SuperCalc worksheet

The worksheet cursor is displayed in inverse video (e.g., black on white instead of white on black) on many terminals, but your terminal may use underlines, carets or brackets in boldface. In any case, there will be some indication that the cursor is in cell A1 at the top left of the display. More about cursors and how to move them later.

## ACTIVE CELL AND CURSOR MOVEMENT

SuperCalc allows you to create a large grid in the computer's memory called a *worksheet*. The entire grid is divided into 63 columns labeled A through BK, and 254 rows labeled 1 through 254. Since there are 26 rather than 63 letters in the alphabet, the twenty-seventh column is labeled AA, the twenty-eighth is AB, and so on. The sixty-third column is labeled BK. The intersections of columns and rows are called *cells*. For instance, in Figure 4.3 the cursor (white box) is in cell A1; that is, column A and row 1. If it were in column C and row 5, it would be in cell C5. If it were in column J and row 200, it would be in cell J200. The cell where the cursor is located is called the *current* or *active* cell. Again, in Figure 4.3, the active cell is A1. The active cell will vary as you change locations on the worksheet.

How is the active cell changed and how do you move from one place to another on the worksheet? Glad you asked! The cursor is the secret of getting from one place to another, and it is moved easily. Look at your keyboard. If you have arrow keys pointing up, down, left and right, these are the *cursor control keys*. From now on these will simply be called *up arrow*, *down arrow*, *right arrow* and *left arrow*. If you don't have specially marked keys, you may have to use your *control* key (usually labeled **CTRL**) and the **E**, **S**, **D** and **X** keys to move the cursor. To do this, hold down the control key and, at the same time, press the correct key to move in the desired direction. The directions and corresponding keys are

up=**E**
down=**X**
right=**D**
left=**S**

In this book, we will use CTL to indicate the control key. So, to move the cursor to the right, hold down the control key and press the **D** key. Try moving the cursor around. When you have the hang of it, return the cursor to A1. Remember, if your system has arrow keys, you do not need to use the control keys to move the cursor; just press the arrow key that points in the direction you want to go. (You can, of course, use the control keys to move the cursor if you prefer.) Generally, when you hold down an arrow key, the cursor will continue to move until you release the key or until the cursor reaches the boundary of the worksheet.

## YOUR WINDOW ON THE WORKSHEET WORLD

The computer stores the entire worksheet in memory, but it can only display part of it on the screen at any one time. The portion of the worksheet you can see is called a *window*. The window in Figure 4.3 has nine columns (A-H) and 20 rows (1-20). The boundaries of that window are cell A1 in the upper righthand corner and cell H20 in the lower lefthand corner. It is important to remember that the window is only a small part of the entire worksheet. Your display or window may be larger or smaller than the one in Figure 4.3, but the great majority of systems will use the window size shown in Figure 4.3.

### Status, Prompt, and Entry Lines

There are several things on your blank worksheet that need to be explained. Notice first that there are three lines at the bottom of the screen:

**>A1**
**Width: 9 Memory: 30 Last Col/Row: A1 ? for Help**
**1>**

The top line is called the *status line* (**>A1**). The status line gives you information about the current state of the worksheet. It also tells you which cell is the *active cell* (the cell that contains the cursor). In Figure 4.3 the active cell is A1. Notice the symbol to the left of **A1**? It may be >, <, ∧ or ∨. This symbol indicates the current direction in which the cursor will move automatically. If you press [RET], the cursor will move in the direction of the symbol. For example, press the right arrow key. The cursor should move to B1 if it was in A1. Now press [RET] several times. Each time [RET] is pressed, the cursor moves in the direction of the right arrow symbol. This feature is handy when entering lots of data in a sequence of cells. You can change the direction of the cursor at any time by pressing one of the arrow keys.

The status line

**<M30**

indicates the active cell is M30 and the cursor movement direction is to the left.

### Prompt Line

The middle line at the bottom of the screen is called the *prompt line*. It contains various types of information. The **Width** message tells you how wide the current column is. Each column on the screen is 9 spaces wide when SuperCalc starts working. That width is suitable for many applications, yet small enough to let you see quite a bit of the worksheet in one window. However, column width can be changed. You can tell SuperCalc to make any column of cells wider or narrower than the original 9 spaces. You can also tell SuperCalc to change the width of all columns in the entire worksheet. However, the larger the column width, the fewer columns you will be able to see in the display window. You will learn how to change column width later. In the following prompt line, the width of the current column has been set to 12 spaces.

**Width: 12 Memory: 33 Last Col/ Row: A1 ? for Help**

The next piece of information on the prompt line is **Memory**. The number refers to the number of kilobytes of memory left for you to use. A *byte* of memory can hold one character. A kilobyte is 1024 bytes or characters. If your system has 64K (K refers to kilobytes) of memory, that means it can hold over 64,000 characters. In the prompt line of the example, memory is 33. That means there are about 33,000 bytes of space left in memory to be used by the worksheet before you run out of memory. Are you wondering why you have a 64K system, but only 33K available to use in SuperCalc? The SuperCalc program and CP/M both take up memory space. The 33K refers to the memory left after you load CP/M and SuperCalc into memory.

The third item, **Last Col/Row: A1**, tells you the last cell you used. The last cell used is not necessarily the active cell. It is the last cell you worked with (e.g., entered data into).

The last item, **? for Help** is the Answer Key* reminder. Any time you're confused or not sure what to do, just press the ? and you will get information about things you might want to do. More about this feature later.

### Entry Line

The bottom line is the entry line, so named because this is where you enter information to be displayed on the worksheet. Notice that the line looks like this:

**1>**

The number 1 indicates the number of the character that is about to be entered. An example will help explain. Use the arrow keys to move the cursor to cell A1 (if it isn't there already). Then type

**S**

What happened? The number changed to a two (2). Now type

**U**

Notice that the number changed to a three (3). Now type

**M**

Again, the number increased by one. This lets you know the number of characters you have entered into the cell. You have entered three letters, and at this point your entry line should look like this:

**4>SUM**

* Answer Key is a trademark of Sorcim Corporation.

The number four tells you that you have entered three characters and the next character will be the fourth.

With your three letter word on the entry line, press [RET]. You should get a message at the extreme righthand side of the status line so that the line now looks like this:

**A1>** **FORMULA ERROR**

How did that happen and what does it mean? A formula error means that you told SuperCalc something it doesn't understand. Formula errors occur only in the entry line. It means that for some reason, the program doesn't understand the three letter entry **SUM**. And you thought this thing was supposed to be so smart! Well, it is – if you learn to speak to it on its own terms.

SuperCalc expects three types of entry: text (letters), data (numbers) and formulas (directions for calculation). When you type in text, it *must* be preceded by quotation marks ("). It is not necessary to put quotation marks at the end of your entry. In fact, if you do, they will be treated as part of the entry and will be included in the cell with your text. Before you try it, use the back arrow key to move the cursor back over to the S. (At this point, the left and right arrow keys can be used to move about on the entry line). Now type

**"SUM**

You can simply type over the existing material; the new material will replace it. Before pressing [RET], your entry line should look like this:

**5>"SUM**

Now press [RET]. Several things should have happened. First, your display should look similar to the one shown in Figure 4.4.

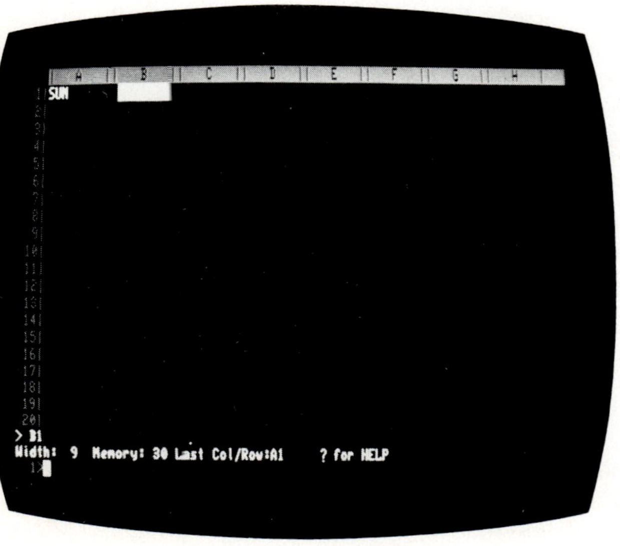


**Figure 4.4** An example of text entry

Where is the cursor? If the direction symbol on the status line was pointing to the left or up, the cursor will still be in cell A1 since it can't move up or to the left. Use your arrow keys (or the control keys) to move the active cell to B1. Now look at the status line. It has changed to read:

**>B1**

That is now your active cell. Nothing else on the worksheet has changed at this point, but just to examine what you've done, press the left arrow key once to move the cursor back to A1.

Do you have the letters **UM** and the cursor in A? What happened to the **S**? It's there. With the right arrow key, move the cursor over one cell (press the key once). Did your **S** appear? On some terminals, the first letter in text may be obscured when the cursor is in that cell. But don't worry, when the cursor is moved in any direction, that first letter will show up.

What else changed on your worksheet? Look at the status line (third line from the bottom); there is a new classification. When the cursor is in A1 the message **Text="SUM** tells you what was entered. This tells you that the material entered in cell A1 was text (as opposed to numbers or formulas) and that the text was **SUM**. Everything else stayed the same; until, that is, you moved the cursor to the right.

Now, you are ready to enter numeric data (numbers). When you enter numeric data, you do not begin with quotation marks. If you do, your entry will be treated as text and not as data. Since text can't be added, subtracted, multiplied or divided, you want to be sure SuperCalc treats your data as numbers and not as text. Now use cell B1 for this example. When the cursor is in B1, type the following:

**1234**[RET]

Does your screen look like the one in Figure 4.5?

Did your cursor jump to the next cell (C1)? If not, use the arrow keys to move the cursor to C1. Notice the status line indicates the active cell is C1, where the cursor is now located. This time the prompt line also changed. It should look like this:

**Width: 9 Memory: 30 Last Col/Row: B1 ? for Help**

The **Last Col/Row** changed from **A1** to **B1** because you entered something in B1. It was the last column and row you used. Move the cursor back to B1 by pressing the back arrow key.

The first thing you may notice is that the digit four is missing. Remember that on some terminals the first letter of text doesn't show up when the cursor is present? Well, when you enter numbers, it's the last digit that seems to vanish. Use the right

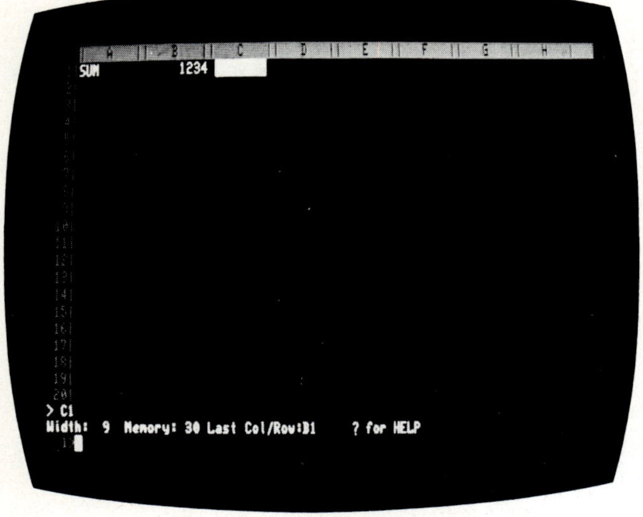


**Figure 4.5** An example of data entry

arrow key to move one column to the right to check this (return the cursor to B1 by pressing the left arrow key).

Look at A1 and notice that the letters start on the far lefthand side of the column. This is called *left justification*. However, the numbers in B1 have five blank spaces in front of them and are on the extreme right side of the column. This is called *right justification*. Text is automatically left-justified and numbers are automatically right-justified unless you tell SuperCalc you want to do it differently.

The other changes are in the bottom lines again. For example, the status line tells you three things. First, the < indicates that the direction of the cursor is to the left. If you press [RET], the cursor will move to A1. Remember when you entered the numbers 1234 and the cursor moved to C1? Then you moved it back to B1. Moving the cursor back manually set the direction to the left. Try this: with the cursor in B1, press the down arrow key to move to B2. What happened to the arrow on the status line? It should now be a down arrow. Press [RET]. The cursor moved down automatically. How do you get back to B1? Press the up arrow. You can change the direction of the cursor at any time. Just remember that changing it means that pressing [RET] will cause the cursor to move in the same direction as the arrow on the status line. Of course, if you don't like the direction you can always change it. Also, if you would rather not have the cursor move automatically on [RET], you can disable this feature completely. Play around with the cursor to get a feel for how it works. After your spin around the spreadsheet, come on back and look at the rest of the status line. Put the cursor in cell B1.

The other information on the status line indicates that the active cell is B1, that you have entered numbers or formulas and that the actual entry was 1234. Any time the word **Form** (short for Formula) appears on the status line, either numbers or an algebraic formula that produces a numeric answer have been entered.

Now move the cursor to C1 and enter

**2456**[RET]

Then move the cursor to D1 and enter the following:

**B1+C1**[RET]

Now things are happening. The entry in C1 was another numeric entry. Then in D1, you entered a simple formula. It instructs SuperCalc to add the numbers in B1 and C1 together and put the answer in D1. You should now have the number 3690 in cell D1. If you move the cursor to D1, note that the status line shows you the formula (B1+C1) while the cell D1 displays the answer to the formula. The ability to write formulas that SuperCalc can use to automatically calculate results is a major feature of the program.

Let's see how this works. If you change the value in C1, the value in D1 should also change. Move the cursor to C1 and enter

**2556**[RET]

The value in D1 is now 3790. The program changed the amount in D1 automatically when you changed the amount in C1.

## EDITING

SuperCalc has a number of features that allow you to correct and modify data as you enter it. Move the cursor to cell C6. Now type the following:

**MISTEEAK**

Don't press the [RET] key yet. You now have some errors on the entry line. First, the quotation marks were omitted at the beginning of this text entry. Let's fix that first. Use the left arrow key to move the cursor over to the **M**. Now press the up arrow key. A space should appear in front of the **M**. Type the " marks there. Now use the right arrow key to move the cursor over to the first **E**. Press the down arrow key twice. That should delete the two **E**s. Finally, move the cursor over to the space after **K** and type **E**. The right and left arrow keys let you move around on the entry line.

The down arrow deletes the letter under the cursor and the up arrow inserts a space so you can add a character. Unless you are a very good typist you will find yourself using these keys often.

If you make a mistake and don't catch it before you press the RET key, SuperCalc will enter the error into a cell. You must then use the EDIT command to correct it. Assume that you do not want **MISTAKE** in C6. Type the following:

**/E**

EDIT is a SuperCalc command which has several options. Since it is a command you must type a / to indicate a command will follow. Then you type an **E** to indicate the command to be used is EDIT.

SuperCalc will respond with

**From? Enter cell**
**/Edit (into current cell),**

SuperCalc wants you to specify the cell which contains the material to be modified or corrected. Type

**C6**RET

SuperCalc will retrieve the material in C6 and display it on the entry line. You can now correct it using the arrow keys to move the cursor and to delete and insert characters. Change "MISTAKE to "MY MISTAKE. When you are finished press the RET key. Cell C6 should now contain the words **MY MISTAKE**.

The EDIT command can be used to modify the contents of any cell on the display. You can even bring in material from one cell and send it to another cell. Just give SuperCalc the name of the source cell when it asks **From?** The edited material will be placed in whatever cell is the active cell as indicated on the status line. If you simply type a comma when SuperCalc asks **From?** it will assume you want to modify the contents of the current active cell. Thus, in the example used above, typing a comma would have had the same effect as typing C6. One more thing about the EDIT command. When you finish your editing, it is not necessary to move the cursor to the end of the line. SuperCalc will enter all the material on the line into a cell no matter where the cursor is located when you press RET.

## SUMMARY

A lot of preliminary information has been covered in this chapter. In Chapter 5 you will learn how to make SuperCalc sit up and do tricks for you, like saving material, deleting, inserting, moving, copying, and so on. Before going on to the next chapter, you may want to take a few minutes to review what has been discussed already.

Below are a few questions for you to answer in order to see how much you've absorbed. This isn't a test: it's just a chance for you to make sure you understand the basics of the worksheet. The page numbers in parentheses after each question indicate where the answer lies. If you can answer all the questions, go on to Chapter 5. If, on the other hand, some things are still unclear, go back and review those topics. Practice, practice, practice.

- How are diskettes loaded? (15)
- What is a prompt? (16)
- What is a cursor? (16)
- What do you type in to get SuperCalc loaded from diskette into your computer's memory? (16)
- When is RET used? (16)
- What is the maximum number of rows and columns? (17)
- What is the active or current cell? (17)
- How is the cursor moved? (17)
- What is a *window* in SuperCalc? (17)
- What is the status line and what information is found there? (18)
- What is the prompt line and what does it tell you? (18)
- What is the entry line? (18)
- What is a formula error? (19)
- Where does a formula error occur and on what line will it appear? (19)
- When must you use a quotation mark in entering information on the worksheet? (19)
- Is a quotation mark necessary for entering numbers? (19)
- How do you edit material on the entry line or in a cell? (20-21)

Chapter 5

# Your Wish is SuperCalc's Command

The title of this chapter may be a little trite, but it's true. Although not a genie, SuperCalc does take your instructions (*commands* as they are called in SuperCalcese) and perform wonders. In this chapter, you will learn the commands to make SuperCalc produce basic worksheet magic.

In Chapter 4, you learned how to get SuperCalc up and running. This chapter will explain many of the commands available when you use SuperCalc. There are many commands at your disposal, and once you've learned some simple procedures, you'll be able to use all of the available commands.

## SAVE, QUIT AND LOAD

Every time you want to enter the *command mode*, you *must* press the slash mark (/). This is necessary each time you want to use a command. If you have come to this chapter directly from Chapter 4, your display should look like the one shown in Figure 5.1. If you don't have a display on your screen, go through Chapter 4 and set up a worksheet similar to the last one there, or copy the one in Figure 5.1.

Try entering the command mode. Type

/

Your display should now look like Figure 5.1 except that the prompt line should now display the following:

**Enter B,C,D,E,F,G,I,L,M,O,P,Q,R,S,T,U,W,X,Z?**

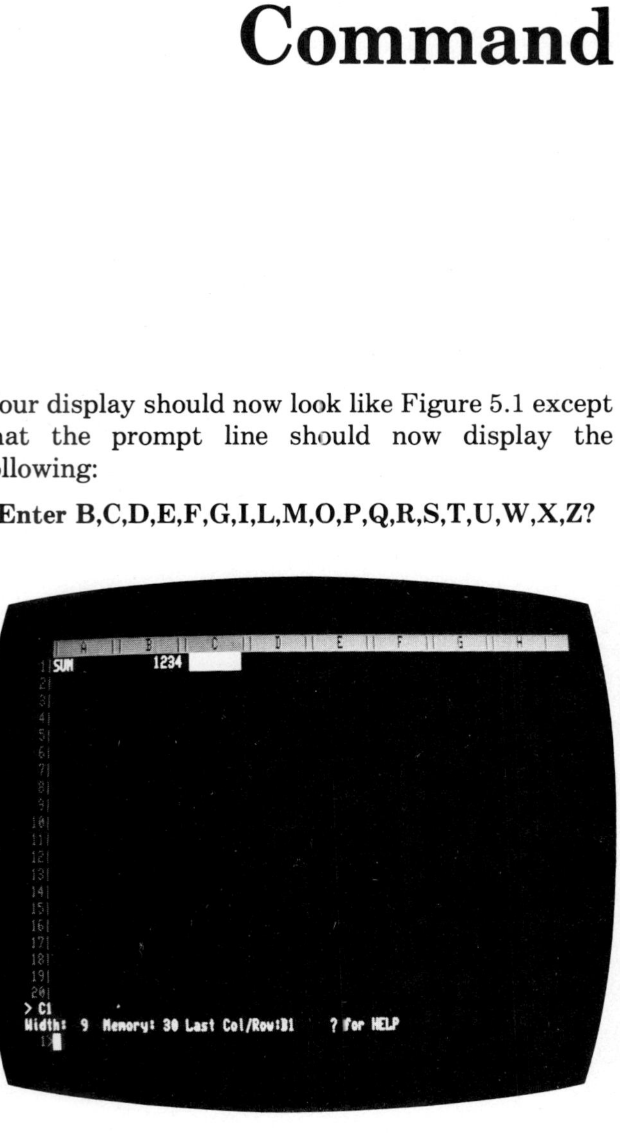


**Figure 5.1** Last worksheet from Chapter Four

What a change! Perhaps now it is a little more clear why it's called the prompt line. All of those letters are prompts for things you can do.

Notice that the prompt line begins with the word **Enter**. Well, that's what you're supposed to do: enter one of those letters. Why? Because each of the letters is an abbreviation for a command. For example, one thing you will want to do is store or save the information you have created. If you've worked for awhile on your worksheet and would like to keep the information you've entered, you can tell the computer to SAVE what's in its memory onto your diskette. Saving is just the reverse of what the computer did when you loaded the SuperCalc program from diskette into the computer. When you save your worksheet on diskette, it is stored for use later. So, SAVE is what you'll do now. Although the worksheet you have may not be the envy of a Harvard MBA, it's a start. After the slash (/), type

**S**

Special Note: It is not necessary to press [RET] when in the command mode. The computer will automatically respond when you press a letter.

Did you see the first part of the magic? All you typed in was an S and the entire word Save and a comma appeared. Does the bottom of your display look like this?

**Enter File Name (or "return" for directory)**
**7>Save,**

Once again, the prompt line changed. You can either enter a file name for your worksheet or look at the directory. A file name is a name you give your work. It can be any combination of numbers and letters up to eight characters long (no spaces or punctuation marks allowed). For now, call this file "Garbage" (it doesn't matter whether you use upper or lower case letters). Type

**Garbage**[RET]

Special Note: It is necessary to press [RET] after typing a file name because the computer has no way of knowing how many characters long your name will be. Remember, [RET] tells the computer that you have finished giving information and that it's time to do something.

Once again, the prompt line has changed. It should look like this:

**A(ll), V(alues), or P(art)?**

There will be times when you'll want to save only particular parts of your worksheet, but those applications will be discussed in later chapters. For present purposes, type

**A**

You need not press [RET].

While the computer was saving your worksheet, did you notice the message **Saving** in the prompt line? Not only does it grant your command, but it tells you when it's doing it! After completing the command, your screen should have returned to the display in Figure 5.1.

What if you don't want to keep your worksheet? Suppose you just want to quit. You can do that, too. As always, first you must type the command symbol. Type

/

You need not press [RET]. This is the last time we'll mention that is it not necessary to press [RET] in the command mode. If you press it out of habit, nothing earth shattering will happen; it's just not necessary.

Now, what you want to do is quit. SuperCalc is fairly versatile in its understanding of English (S for SAVE), and will respond appropriately when you use Q for QUIT. Try it. After the slash, type

**Q**

Your system should have responded with:

**EXIT SuperCalc? Y(es) or N(o)**

Notice too, that the word Quit was spelled out (this will happen with each of the command choices). If you've changed your mind and don't want to quit, SuperCalc will let you; just type the letter **N** for N(o). For demonstration purposes, type

**Y**

You should now have a totally blank screen except for a lonely prompt (**A>**) in the upper lefthand corner. You are now out of the SuperCalc program and back using CP/M. Now is a good time to refresh your memory on how to get the program started and how to load in the worksheet called "Garbage". Type

**SC**[RET]

and SuperCalc should be loaded into memory again and be ready to go. Now press [RET]. Assuming you have SuperCalc loaded and you are looking at a blank worksheet, you can now load the file "Garbage". LOAD is a command and must therefore by summoned by the command symbol. Type

/

As you might have guessed, the letter for LOAD is L, so type

**L**

Your screen should now resemble the following:

**Enter File Name (or "return" for directory)**
**7>/Load,**

Because you saved a file, you can now load it from the diskette into the computer's memory. To do that, type

**Garbage** RET

The prompt line now reads

**A(ll or P(art)?**

Since this worksheet is small, go ahead and ask for all of it by typing:

**A**

Again, watch as the prompt line lets you know what's happening. Remember that when you saved "Garbage" it reported: **Saving**. This time it should read:

**Loading,**

When that disappears, you should see the same worksheet as in Figure 5.1.

Now you can load, save and quit. You have within your control three of the 19 commands used in SuperCalc, perhaps the three most crucial. There's plenty more to go, but you should feel confident that you have mastered important information already.

## ANSWER KEY

With 19 commands at your disposal, what if you don't know the best one to choose, or you don't know what the letters stand for, or you forget? Help is always available. Remember in Chapter 4 the Answer Key (?) was mentioned? It works in two ways: First, you can get general information about how to use SuperCalc. Type

**?**

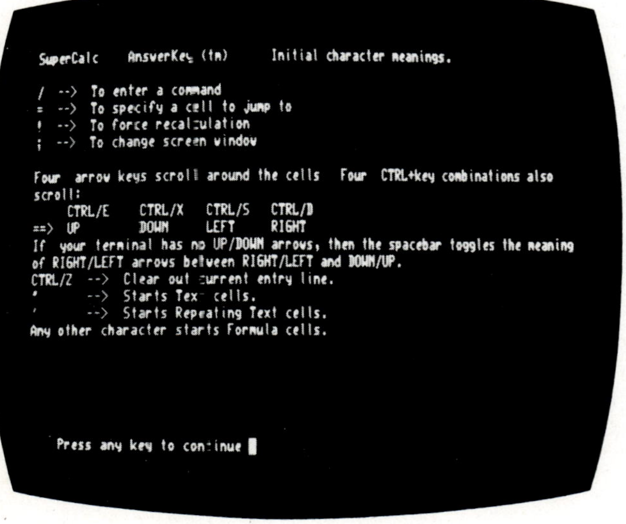
SuperCalc AnswerKey (tm) Initial character meanings.
/ --> To enter a command
= --> To specify a cell to jump to
! --> To force recalculation
; --> To change screen window
Four arrow keys scroll around the cells Four CTRL+key combinations also scroll:
CTRL/E CTRL/X CTRL/S CTRL/D
==> UP DOWN LEFT RIGHT
If your terminal has no UP/DOWN arrows, then the spacebar toggles the meaning of RIGHT/LEFT arrows between RIGHT/LEFT and DOWN/UP.
CTRL/Z --> Clear out current entry line.
" --> Starts Text cells.
' --> Starts Repeating Text cells.
Any other character starts Formula cells.
Press any key to continue

**Figure 5.2** The Answer Key

Most of the items in Figure 5.2 have already been discussed, but a few haven't. The ones that aren't familiar, such as

**"= –> To specify a cell to jump to"**
**"! –> To force a recalculation"**

will be explained in later sections where they are used in examples.

The second way the ? is used is to find out more about commands. For this purpose, it must be preceded by the slash. Press any key to return to the worksheet, then type

**/**

You should have a screen like the one in Figure 5.3 which tells you three things about each command.

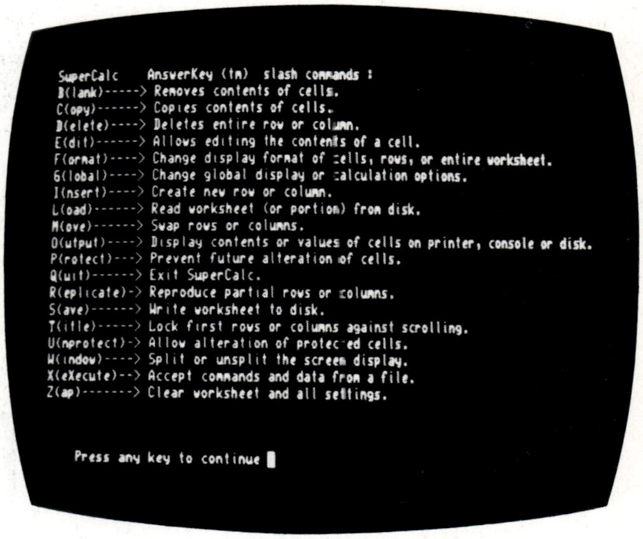
SuperCalc AnswerKey (tm) slash commands :
B(lank)-----> Removes contents of cells.
C(opy)------> Copies contents of cells.
D(elete)----> Deletes entire row or column.
E(dit)------> Allows editing the contents of a cell.
F(ormat)----> Change display format of cells, rows, or entire worksheet.
G(lobal)----> Change global display or calculation options.
I(nsert)----> Create new row or column.
L(oad)------> Read worksheet (or portion) from disk.
M(ove)------> Swap rows or columns.
O(utput)----> Display contents or values of cells on printer, console or disk.
P(rotect)---> Prevent future alteration of cells.
Q(uit)------> Exit SuperCalc.
R(eplicate)-> Reproduce partial rows or columns.
S(ave)------> Write worksheet to disk.
T(itle)-----> Lock first rows or columns against scrolling.
U(nprotect)-> Allow alteration of protected cells.
W(indow)----> Split or unsplit the screen display.
X(eXecute)--> Accept commands and data from a file.
Z(ap)-------> Clear worksheet and all settings.
Press any key to continue

**Figure 5.3** The command Answer Key

First, it lists each single letter. Second, it tells what the letter stands for. And third, a brief description of the command is given. For example, you know that L stands for LOAD and that it means you can retrieve information stored on diskette and put it in the computer's memory. If at any time you forget or are uncertain about a command, all you have to do is type the command symbol (/) and the question mark to find out more about it.

The usefulness of the Answer Key does not end here. In addition to getting general information on all of the commands, you can use the ? to get specific details on each of the commands. Press any key to get back to the worksheet and try an example. Type a slash if one isn't displayed on the entry line. Your prompt and entry line should be similar to this:

**Enter B,C,D,E,F,G,I,L,M,O,P,Q,R,S,T,U,W,X,Z,?**
**2>/**

## OUTPUT

Suppose you have a worksheet full of information that you are going to need at a meeting in Dallas next week. How can you get all of that hard work to the meeting? You could ship your computer to Dallas, but sending such sensitive equipment can be tricky. Another alternative is to get a printout or *hard copy* of your worksheet and take it with you. Since a hard copy is important to your use of the program, this will serve as an example of the specific details provided by the Answer Key.

Earlier it was stated that SuperCalc is "understanding" in its use of the English language (L for LOAD, S for SAVE, etc.). There are several likely candidates for getting a printout. P might be one. Try it. Type

**P**

Do your prompt and entry lines look like this?

**Enter Range**
**10>/Protect,**

That has nothing to do with printing, so that was not the right choice (PROTECT will be discussed later). Now you have information on the entry line you don't want. Any time you change your mind, or make a mistake on the entry line, press the back arrow key to erase what you don't want. To remove the **Protect,** press the back arrow once. That should erase everything except the command symbol /.

Now, back to the task at hand. What might be another possibility to get a hard copy of the material? How about H for HARDCOPY? There isn't an H? When all else fails, use the Answer Key. To find out what SuperCalc accepts as a printing command, enter

**/?**

You may have to read the explanation of each command to find the print command. In doing so, you will probably run across several words and concepts that have little, if any, meaning to you at this point. Don't worry, you'll soon know what each command does. Anyway, when you reach O(UTPUT), you have found it. The definition, "Display contents or values of cells on printer, console, or disk," means getting a printout or viewing it on the display screen or putting it on disk. Regardless of the tangled mess of words, OUTPUT is what you want. Again, get back to the worksheet by pressing any key.

So, OUTPUT will give you a hard copy of your worksheet. Go another step and type

**O**

Your prompt line should read:

**D(isplay) or C(ontents) report?**

What does this mean? To find out, use the Answer Key. Type

**?**

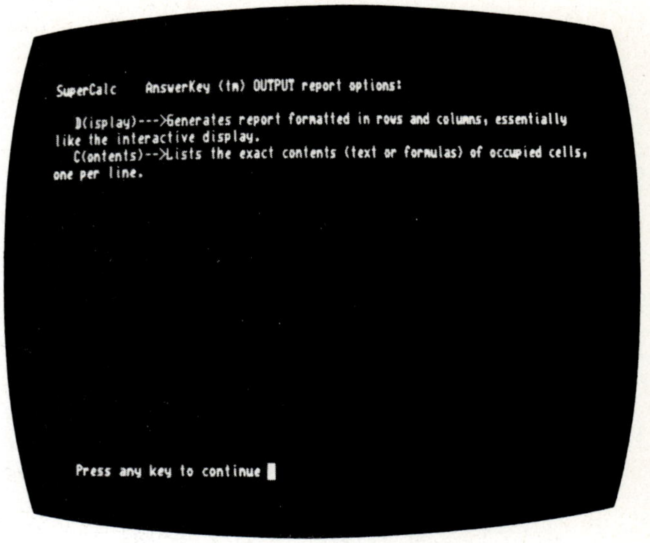


**Figure 5.4** The Answer Key explains Display and Contents for the OUTPUT command

A new screen, like the one shown in Figure 5.4, should appear and give you specific information on Display and Contents. In short, Display will show your work in the same format as on the worksheet. The outcome of a formula is displayed instead of the formula itself. Contents, on the other hand, prints out what you entered in each cell – either text or formulas. When you are ready, press any key to return to the worksheet.

Once you have decided whether you want a Display or Contents printout, you can indicate your decision. For now, request a Display by typing:

**D**

The prompt line changes (again) to

**Enter Range**

What does range mean? Press the Answer Key to see. Your display looks like the one shown in Figure 5.5.

Unfortunately, SuperCalc's explanation of range in the Help section is a little confusing. In addition, early versions of the documentation that comes with your SuperCalc program use the term "block" in more than one way. Here are our definitions of the terms used in SuperCalc:

*Range.* SuperCalc uses this term as a general, umbrella label for anything that tells SuperCalc what part of the worksheet is to be acted upon. When it asks for a range you can specify one cell (e.g., K21), several cells (K21, K26, A34), a series of cells (A1:A5

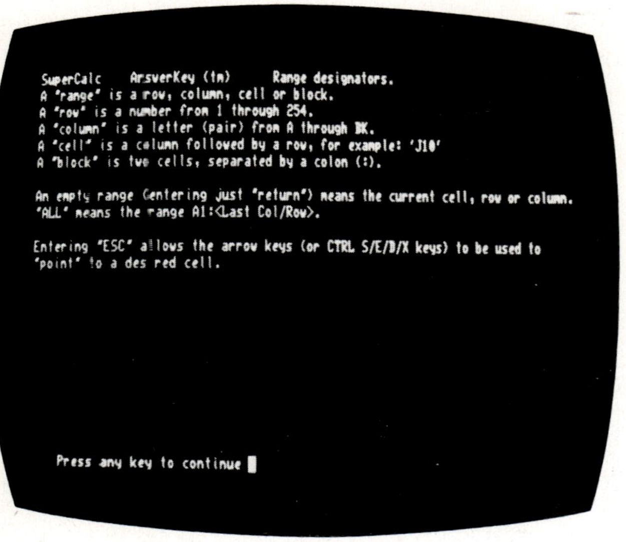


**Figure 5.5** The Answer Key explains Range

–that is shorthand for A1, A2, A3, A4, and A5) and even a block of cells. Block will be dealt with later. All the examples above are considered a range by SuperCalc. Many of the commands will accept any of them as a range. However, some commands accept some types of ranges but not others. Let's look at the different types of ranges.

*Cell.* A cell has already been defined. It is the basic element in the worksheet and is specified by one or two letters (the column designation) and a number (the row designation). A1, BE55, C48 and R21 are all valid cell designations. In addition to the standard way of designating a cell, some SuperCalc commands let you press the [RET] key to indicate the active cell when responding to a request for a range. If a command asks for a specific cell, a row, or a column, you can also type a comma (,). If your active cell is C4, typing a comma is the same as typing C4 if a cell designation is required, or C if a column designation is needed, or 4 if a row is to be identified.

Finally, the **ESCAPE** key can also be used to designate a cell. If you press the **ESCAPE** key, the entry line will change. Wherever the cursor was located when you pressed the **ESCAPE** key, that cell becomes the current or active cell. The **ESCAPE** key is thus a shorthand way of designating the active cell. In addition, if you press the **ESCAPE** key and then use the cursor keys to move around on the worksheet, the active cell listed on the entry line and the status line will change. When you enter a comma (,) or [RET], that cell will be used in the command. That means you can change the cell to be acted upon by some commands if you use **ESCAPE** to designate the active cell. You may want to experiment with the use of the **ESCAPE** key after completing this lesson.

*Row.* A row is defined by a number from 1 to 254.

*Column.* A column is defined by one or two letters from A to BK.

*Block.* The SuperCalc definition of a block, "two cells, separated by a colon," explains how you can specify a block. There are actually two types of blocks. One type specifies a sequence of cells located next to each other in the same row or column. For example, A1:A4 is a block that includes cells A1, A2, A3, and A4. The block A1:D1 is a block that includes cells A1, B1, C1, and D1.

Another type of block is specified by A1:D4. Look at the diagram below.

| | | | |
|---|---|---|---|
| A1 | B1 | C1 | D1 |
| A2 | B2 | C2 | D2 |
| A3 | B3 | C3 | D3 |
| A4 | B4 | C4 | D4 |

The block A1:D4 specifies all sixteen cells in the diagram above. A1 defines the top left border of the block, and D4 defines the bottom right border of the block. This type of block can be used to change or modify large segments of the worksheet with one command entry. Note that A1:D1 is a block made up of the top row of cells, A1:A4 is the left row of cells, D1:D4 is the right row of cells, and A1:D4 takes in all the cells.

*List.* A list is a mixed bag of cell designations. Some commands let you specify a range like this: A1,D1:D4,C3. This is a list that includes the cells A1, D1, D2, D3, D4 and C3. Lists are useful when the cells you want to work with are not in one row or column, and do not constitute one complete block.

*All.* All is a range which specifies all the currently active cells in the worksheet. It is useful when displaying or printing a full report of the contents of the spread sheet.

Remember that all of the terms listed above (cell, row, column, block and list) are different types of ranges. If a command asks you for a range, you can generally use any of the types of ranges we have defined (the exceptions are list and all, which are not accepted by a number of SuperCalc commands).

Press any key to get back to the worksheet. Use your back arrow key to erase the OUTPUT command that you've started. Because your worksheet is almost blank, defining a range will have little meaning. In order to better understand range, you need to enter some material in various locations on your worksheet. Use the arrow keys to move to C1 and enter

**5678[RET]**

Now, in D1 enter

**"sample[RET]**

Notice how the s in D1 is against the 8 in C1. That is because numbers are right-justified and text is left-justified. In E1, enter

**"worksheet[RET]**

Now, use the back arrow key to move back to column A and the down arrow to move to row 10. Your active cell (where the cursor is located) should now be A10. Enter

**"This[RET]**

If you followed the directions above to move your cursor, then the cursor is set to move down and has jumped to A11. You will need to use the up arrow key to get it back to A10 and the right arrow key to move to B10. In B10 enter

**"is[RET]**

In C10

**"a[RET]**

In D10

**"test[RET]**

Your worksheet should now look like the one in Figure 5.6.

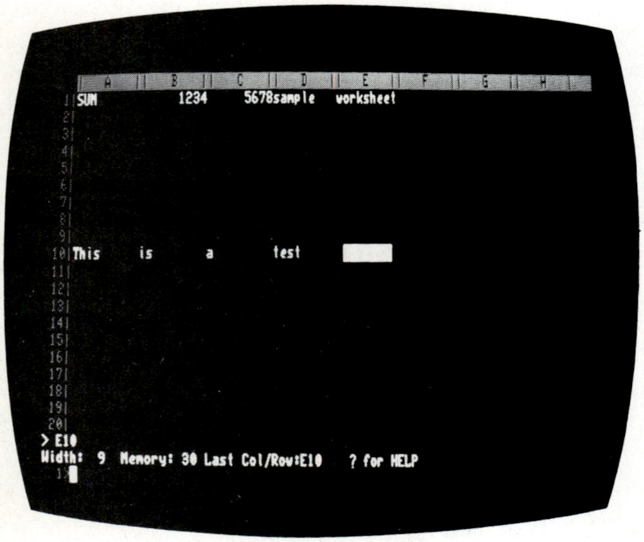


**Figure 5.6** Revised worksheet

Back to the task at hand – trying out Range. After entering material on the worksheet, it is again necessary to set up for OUTPUT on the entry line. Because there is no need to press [RET] after commands, the sequence of /, OUTPUT and Display can be entered one right after the other. Type

**/OD**

Now the prompt line asks for Range. Range, for this command, is a cell, row, column or block. To specify a range enter

**A1:E10[RET]**

The range you specified includes all cells, rows and columns from A1 in the upper right corner to E10 in the lower left corner. This is also a block since it extends across several rows and columns. Remember that a block is one type of range.

Wouldn't it be nice if you could see how the range looks before it's printed out? Well, SuperCalc thought about that, too. To see how A1:E10 will look when it is printed, you can use the Console option from the prompt line (console simply means your screen). Type

**C**

Your screen should now resemble Figure 5.7, which also looks a lot like Figure 5.6, the worksheet. Any output from Display will result in a product that is formatted to look like the display of the worksheet.

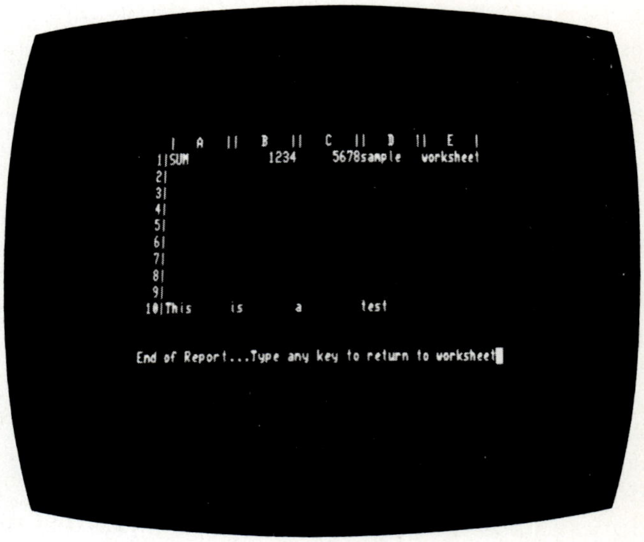


**Figure 5.7** Console display of worksheet

Press any key to get back the worksheet and we'll try some other range options. Remember to start the OUTPUT sequence by entering

**/OD**

which will set the OUTPUT command with the Display option.

This time, instead of entering a block for a range, enter a single column such as

**B[RET]**

Then, to view your range, choose the Console option by entering

**C**

Your display should now look like the one in Figure 5.8.

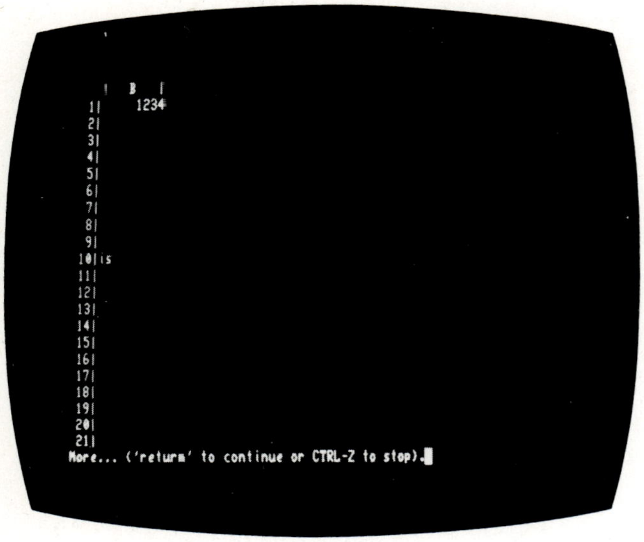


**Figure 5.8** Console display of column B

If you press the [RET] key it will show you more of column B even though there is no data in any cell below B10. The computer has no way of knowing that you really only wanted to see column B from B1 to B10. All that was specified was column B. The bottom of the screen reads

**More....('return' to continue or CTRL-Z to stop).**

This means there are more lines than can be displayed at one time; if you want to see them, press [RET]. Do that to see what happens. You will see more rows and the same message at the bottom of the screen. You can either press [RET] to see more blank rows or use [CTL]-**Z**. ([CTL] stands for the control key.) Press the control key and the **Z** key at the same time to get back to the worksheet.

Return to the worksheet, type **/OD** again and then type in the following range:

**A1:E10**[RET]

Still the prompt line changes to ask more questions! Your prompt line should read

**Enter Device: P(rinter), S(etup), C(onsole), or D(isk)**

Setup and Disk will be discussed later; right now let's do some printing. Be sure your printer is plugged in, turned on and correctly connected to the computer. Then type

**P**

and listen to your printer do its thing! (If you don't have a printer, use the C option instead of P and the material will be displayed on the screen.)

If you select the P option and there is no printer connected, or if the printer is improperly connected, SuperCalc may "lock up." That is, it may refuse to respond to any of your instructions. If this happens, you may want to take your diskettes out of the disk drives, turn everything off, and then start over. When SuperCalc tries to print something it will look to see if the printer is sending a "ready" signal before beginning. If the printer is not on, there will be no ready signal and SuperCalc may simply wait until it gets one. That, of course, would be forever if the printer isn't on. Sometimes it is only necessary to switch the printer on to "unlock" SuperCalc. Then you can press the [CTL] and **Z** keys to stop printing. Let's assume everything went according to plan, however. Your printout is shown in Figure 5.9. After you've stopped beaming at your first SuperCalc printout, take a look at the prompt line. It tells you that the printing is finished (that's what **End of Report** means). If you press any key, you will return to your worksheet.

```
         A           B           C        D         E
 1 SUM              1234        5678sample    worksheet
 2
 3
 4
 5
 6
 7
 8
 9
10 This      is         a           test
```

**Figure 5.9** Printout of sample worksheet (Display)

In addition, the status line has a different message. This message is displayed just before printing begins, during printing and after the printer has stopped. The prompt line should read

**CTRL-Z to STOP print**

This means that if you want to stop the printing process, you can press the [CTL] (control) key and the **Z** key at the same time and the printer will stop.

If your printer didn't print, make sure it's plugged in, connected to the computer and turned on. If all that checks out, go back and make sure you followed the directions carefully. If there is an error at some point on the entry line, an error message will appear on the status line. If everything has been entered properly and all connections between the computer, printer and source of electricity are fine, call your dealer and ask for help.

Now that you know the basics of printing using the Display option, take a look at the Contents option. Remember that the Display option prints the worksheet in the same format as it normally appears. The Contents option is somewhat different.

Since you have just used the printer, you will need to begin the OUTPUT command again. Press any key to get back to the worksheet and enter the command symbol (/) and the **O** for OUTPUT:

**/O**

This time, when asked for either Display or Contents, select Contents by typing

**C**

As with the Display option, a range is required. (Remember the meaning of range? If not, use the Answer Key (?) to bring up the definition on the screen.) Use the same range as you did in Display to see how the two options differ. Type

**A1:E10**

Ready to print? Then enter

**P**

Your printout should look like Figure 5.10.

```
SuperCalc ver. B5.04
SUM
A1        = "SUM
B1        = 1234
C1        = 5678
D1        = "sample
E1        = "worksheet
A10        = "This
B10        = "is
C10        = "a
D10        = "test
```

**Figure 5.10** Printout of sample worksheet (Contents)

What are the differences between the Display and Contents printout? It is a little like asking, "Do you want problems listed (e.g., 54+46) or the answers (e.g., 100)?" Content printouts tell you exactly what is in the cells. That is, if you put B1+65 in cell C5, the Content format will show you that B1+65 is in cell C5. The Display format printout would not show B1+65. Instead, it would determine what value is in cell B1, add that value to 65, and display the sum in cell C5. If B1 has a value of 21 then C1 would show the value 86.

In essence, Contents printouts show instructions and Display formats give the solutions to these instructions. On the left side of the Contents printout, cell numbers within the range you specified (A1:E10) are displayed. Notice that while there are other cells within the range (A2-A9, B2-B9, C2-C9, etc.) none of those were printed because they do not contain information. The Contents option is concerned only with those cells that have something in them: the "contents" are printed.

**The Setup Option**

Return to the worksheet and type

**/ODA1:D10**RET
**S**

A new screen with information about Setup has appeared. Setup lets you define several things important to printing. You can change several different printing parameters with this option. Starting at the top, let's change the settings.

*Length of page.* This refers to the number of lines that will be printed on each sheet. How long is your paper? If you use standard 8½×11-inch paper, it will require a different page length than 11⅜×14-inch paper. Type

**L**

The prompt line changes to

**Enter number (0-255), then return**

Let's say you will be printing on standard size paper and want 50 lines per page. Type

**50**RET

The *default* or original length shown at the top of the screen was 66. When you entered 50, it replaced 66. Now each page will be 50 lines long. The prompt line now shows

**L(ength), W(idth), S(etup) or P(rint)?**

*Width of page.* Since you are using standard paper, you don't want the regular or default value of 132 characters in width. To change this setting, type

**W**

Again, enter a value from 0 to 255. This time make it 70, so type

**70**RET

The value under Width at the top of the screen changes from 132 to 70, and the prompt line returns to its previous prompt.

At this point, you have given the computer all the information it needs to start printing. If your printer is plugged into the computer, plugged into electricity and turned on, you can print out your designated block (A1:E10) by typing

**P**

Your printout should resemble the one in Figure 5.11.

There is another option under Setup called Manual Setup Codes. Some printers can be given instructions that modify the way they print. For example, several dot matrix printers can print five or six different sizes of text. Some printers can even be ad-

```
        A          B          C          D          E
 1 SUM             1234       5678sample    worksheet
 2
 3
 4
 5
 6
 7
 8
 9
10 This      is         a          test
```

**Figure 5.11** Setup printout

justed for the quality of the print they produce, from very fast, "draft" quality printouts to slower "correspondence" quality printouts. If you select the S option, SuperCalc will connect the keyboard you are using directly to the printer. Anything you type in will be sent directly to the printer. That means you can send the printer any codes that are required for it to perform as you wish. Since printers vary considerably, we will not provide an example of how S is used. However, if you have one of the "software controllable" printers this option will be worth investigating.

Rather than using Setup to print, you could also have had your worksheet displayed on the screen or console. The Console option lets you see what's going to be printed before you give the command to print. This could be important if, for example, you need to make revisions on the worksheet or on the formulas in the worksheet.

### The Disk Option

There is one more option in OUTPUT, and that is the Disk option. You learned the difference between Display and Contents; you know the different types of range; you can print; you can enter your specific printing needs by using Setup; and you have briefly covered Console. To cover this one last area, set up again for OUTPUT and Display (you could also use Contents; the Disk option works the same way with either one) by typing

**/OD**

Before you enter the range, the difference between OUTPUT with the Disk option and the SAVE command needs to be discussed. Up to now, this procedure is just like the one you use to SAVE, but the procedure is all that is similar. Using the OUTPUT and Disk command stores the contents of your worksheet, but not for use in SuperCalc again. The information stored with this routine is formatted to work with another CP/M program, such as a word processing system. It is not available to SuperCalc if it has been stored through OUTPUT. Perhaps working through an example will help.

Now, for range, enter

**A1:E10** RET

Enter

**D**

to tell the computer you want the Disk option. Now type the following file name:

**MYFILE** RET

Notice that the prompt line did not say it was Saving or "Disking" as you might have expected. There were no clues at all as to what was happening. Now, try to LOAD that file back. First, the command symbol:

**/**

Then the LOAD command:

**L**

Then the file name:

**MYFILE**

The status line reports

**File NOT on Disk**

You have done everything correctly and followed the procedure step by step, but it still isn't there. It isn't supposed to be. This file is not available to SuperCalc. That doesn't mean it's lost! Sometimes you will want information from your worksheet to be worked into, or interfaced with, a word processing program, to be a part of a report, for example. Just remember not to use this method of storing if you want to have access to the material through SuperCalc.

You now have experienced just about everything that can be done with printing or getting output to a printer, console (screen) or disk. You also have used three other commands in addition to OUTPUT: LOAD, SAVE and QUIT. In the next chapter, you will learn most of the commands while setting up an expense account.

## SUMMARY

In this chapter, you have learned how to get started with SuperCalc. The material presented here is essential, so please be sure that you understand it. Here is a list of the things that we covered. Each item is followed by a page number showing where it was first introduced:

| | |
|---|---|
| All | 27 |
| Answer Key | 25 |
| block | 27 |
| cell | 27 |
| column | 27 |

If you are not completely familiar with all of these terms, re-read the sections that are not clear. In addition, you may want to look up the commands in the Reference Section.

# Chapter 6

# SuperCalc and the Expense Account

In this chapter, you will learn how SuperCalc can help you manage your time better. You will use the program to construct an expense account. Hopefully, this will accomplish three things: it will give you an introduction to the SuperCalc command structure; it will give you more practice in entering data; and it will relieve you of the drudgery of doing expense accounts. Throughout this chapter the emphasis is on how to use the program. There will be times when you say to yourself, "I already have a way of doing this and my way seems easier." In some cases you'll be right, but it's important to learn all of the functions of SuperCalc to get the most out of it.

Hopefully, you will learn something else from this chapter . . . *patience*. Worksheet design and construction can be tedious, but it is worth it. Once you have carefully designed and constructed your worksheet, you never have to do it again. However, the first time you do it, it may take you a lot of time. In fact, you will probably find that you could have done it faster manually. This won't be true the second time though. A small time investment the first time can reap enormous rewards later on, so please be patient. In this chapter, you will construct the expense account one piece at a time, but once it is done you'll never have to do it again. Once the worksheet is designed and constructed all you have to do is plug the numbers in.

As you make progress with the program, you will learn easier ways of doing things on your own. In addition, you will learn how to adapt the expense account to your own needs. As you work through this chapter, you may tire of the reminders to save your work. Hopefully, by saving frequently, the process will become second nature to you. You should save your work any time you leave the computer, any time you quit for the day, and any time . . . . That is because it is not uncommon to lose the information in the computer's memory (e.g., a power glitch or outage), but once the material is saved on diskette, it is less likely to be lost.

## SETTING UP THE WORKSHEET

To begin, load SuperCalc into your system (see the Appendix if you need help). When the worksheet comes up, the active cell should be A1 and the direction (according to the status line) should be to the right. If your worksheet is different, please use the arrow keys to set the active cell and direction.

You will now create headings for your expense account. Type

"EXPENSE ACCOUNT FOR (insert your name)[RET]

Using the right arrow, move the worksheet cursor to F1. As you can see, the program displays your text from columns A1 to D1. If your text exceeds the column width, the program will still display it as long as it does not encounter a cell with data in it.

In F1, enter

"WEEK ENDING 5/8/82[RET]

With G1 being the active cell, it looks as though there was not enough room to print all of the above message. Use the right arrow key to move to H1 and the rest of the message appears.

Now, we want to move to A2. The traditional way to do that would be to use the arrow keys, but there is a quicker method. It's called the GO TO command. The symbol for the GO TO command is the equal sign (=). You can specify which cell you want to go to by typing the equal sign (=) and the name of the cell. For example, you now want to go to A2. To do that, type

=

What happened when you entered the =? A right arrow appeared on the entry line. The prompt line changed to read

**Enter cell to jump to.**

Now, enter

A2[RET]

It is easier than pressing the arrow keys all the time, isn't it? And usually a lot faster, too. You don't have to pause between the = and the cell location. For example, if you want to GO TO E10, enter

=E10[RET]

and you'll be there before you know it! You may want to practice this a few times just so you'll remember this easy way to move the cursor. Notice, too, that the direction the cursor will move when you press [RET] (as shown on the status line) is not affected by the GO TO instruction. If its direction was to the left before GO TO, it will still be to the left afterward, even if you moved the cursor in some other direction. When you're finished, return the cursor to A2.

Now that you're in A2, enter

"DAILY EXPENSES[RET]

Notice again that not all of the message seems to be there. Just to be sure it is, use the right arrow key to go to C2. See? It's just like you entered. Ready for another aspect of the GOTO command? Your cursor is now in C2 and you want to go to A3 to enter another category. You could type in =**A3** and get there just fine. But, here's another shorthand tip: any time you want to be in column A, any row, you can merely enter the row number without the column letter. For example, you now want to be in A3. Enter

=3[RET]

and the cursor goes to A3. Remember, this only works when you want to be in column A, but it's handy to know.

Your cursor is in A3 and the direction is to the right. If your worksheet is different from this, please set it before going on.

Before typing in the next set of headings, see if you can predict how the worksheet will look. After you've anticipated the outcome, type

"WEEKDAY[RET]
"DATE[RET]
[RET]
"LOCATION[RET]
"TRANSPT[RET]
"HOTEL[RET]
"ENTERTN[RET]
"MISC.[RET]
"TOTAL[RET]

Did it turn out as you expected? Your worksheet should look like the one in Figure 6.1. Notice that column A has disappeared and that column I is the last column on the right. This process is called *scrolling*. When you change the window (the portion of the worksheet you see) by moving right, left, up, or down, you are scrolling the worksheet. Move the cursor to the right a couple of times and watch the

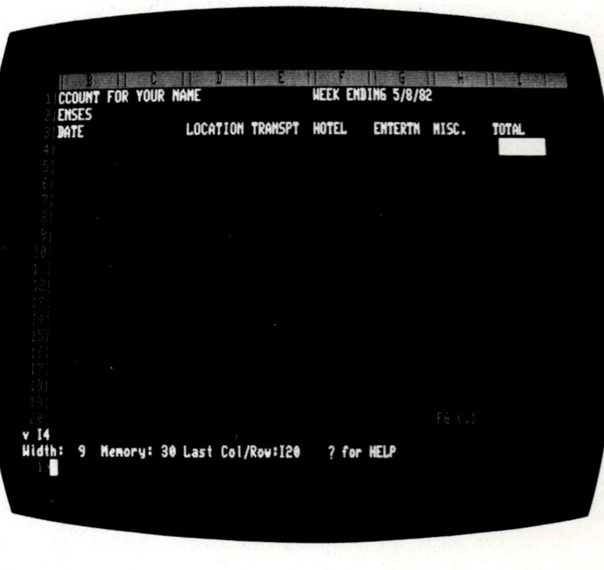


**Figure 6.1** Worksheet headers

columns on the left disappear while more columns appear from the right side of the screen. As you move the cursor back to the left, the columns that had disappeared come back and the columns to the right vanish. You can do the same thing vertically by moving the cursor down. When you get to row 20 and move down one more row, row 1 disappears and row 21 comes up from the bottom. Keep moving down to see how this works. When you're comfortable with scrolling in all directions, use the arrow keys to go back to A5 and make sure the arrow on the status line is pointing down.

Enter another series of headings. Can you predict how the worksheet will look?

**"SUNDAY** [RET]
**"MONDAY** [RET]
**"TUESDAY** [RET]
**"WEDNESDAY** [RET]
**"THURSDAY** [RET]
**"FRIDAY** [RET]
**"SATURDAY** [RET]
**"  TOTAL** [RET]

Be sure to leave two spaces in front of **TOTAL**. Your display should look like the one in Figure 6.2.

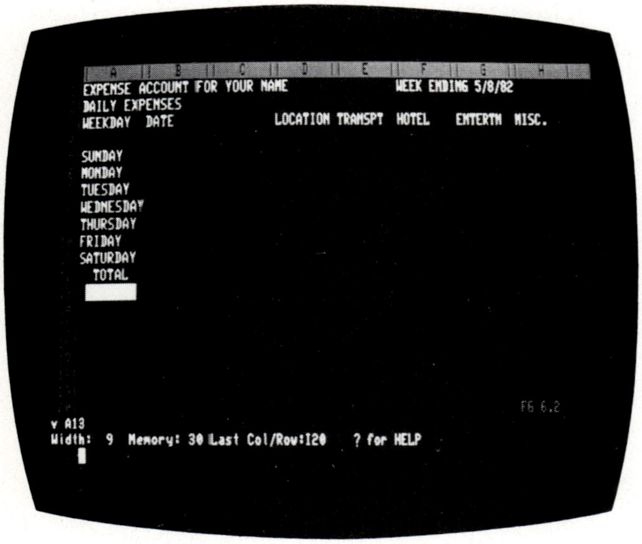


**Figure 6.2** Days of the week

## Replicate Command

Now, you'll enter the month, May, into B5:

**"May** [RET]

You also want the month in each cell from B6 to B11. You could type it in all six times, or you can use the REPLICATE command. The REPLICATE command will copy the contents of one cell into a group of cells. For instance, you could enter May into every cell on the worksheet using the REPLICATE command. The real power of this command is that REPLICATE copies not only numbers and text, but also formulas. This feature will be examined in detail later. For the time being, let's use this command to enter May. Because REPLICATE is a command, it must be preceded by the command symbol (/). Enter

**/R**

The program will respond

**From? (Enter Range)**

To replicate May from cell B5 respond

**B5** [RET]

and the computer will display

**To? (Enter Range), then Return; or "," for Options**

You want May in B5 to B11, so enter

**B6:B11** [RET]

And there is May in all the rows you requested. Your worksheet should now look like the one shown in Figure 6.3.

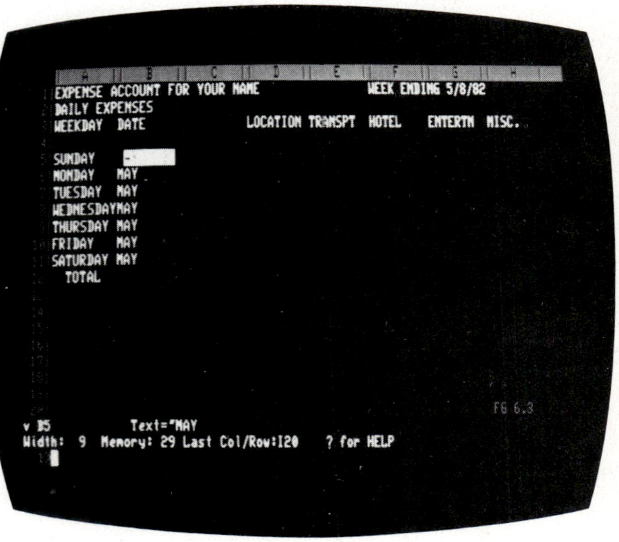


**Figure 6.3** Expense account using Replicate

## Addition

Ready to go for the dates? Make sure C5 is your active cell and the direction of the cursor is down, because you are going to enter a formula that will automatically enter the dates. In cell C5, enter

**2** [RET]

You will see a 2 displayed in cell C5. The cursor should now be in C6. Here you will enter your first formula. This formula computes the date. With the cursor on C6, type

**C5+1**[RET]

The number 3 should appear. In C7, type

**C5+2**[RET]

Did you get a 4? Good! In C8, enter

**C5+3**[RET]

In C9, enter

**C5+4**[RET]

In C10

**C5+5**[RET]

And, finally, in C11, enter

**C5+6**[RET]

Your worksheet should now look like the one in Figure 6.4. The last date should be May 8. It may have been easier to type in the dates, but this process gave you a chance to use a formula—this practice will be very helpful later.

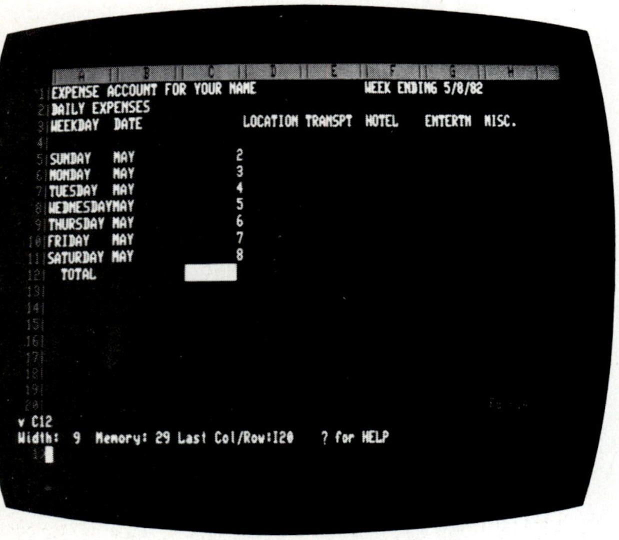


**Figure 6.4** Worksheet with dates

Move your cursor back up to C11. Notice that the status line displays the formula while the worksheet displays the sum of the formula. This is helpful if you find a strange figure in a cell and wonder how in the world it got there. By looking at the status line, you can see if the figure is the solution to a formula. This would be a good time to save your work. Type

**/S**

Remember, you have a diskette in Drive A and one in Drive B. The system diskette is in Drive A, so you'll want to store your worksheet on Drive B. Select a file name. Let's call this one "Expense." Designate the drive to be used and the file name by entering

**B:EXPENSE**[RET]

Also, save the entire worksheet by typing

**A**

in response to the A(ll) or P(art) prompt. If you look quickly at the prompt line, you will notice that it reports it is Saving.

In this book, a standard disk usage convention is assumed: the diskette with CP/M and SuperCalc is always in Drive A and the data diskette is in Drive B. That is a common, easy to learn system. Many SuperCalc users put CP/M and SuperCalc on a diskette, place it in Drive A and then use the rest of the space on that diskette to store their worksheet files (e.g., "Expense" above). They feel having everything on one diskette is more convenient. In any case, it is a good idea to save your work often. Also, it is a good idea to create a second copy of your worksheet on another diskette before you turn the computer off.

### FORMAT Command

As you can see, there is a wide space between the word "May" and the dates. For aesthetic reasons, you would like to put the numbers closer to May. You can do this with the FORMAT command. FORMAT will tell the program to left justify the numbers and/or right justify the text if you'd like. The screen display is normally just the opposite (right-justified numbers and left-justified text). To begin the FORMAT sequence, enter

**/F**

and the computer will respond

**Enter Level: G(lobal), C(olumn), R(ow), or E(ntry)**
**9>/Format,**

You want to format the entry (a cell or group of cells, i.e., column B) so type

**E**

and the computer will respond

**Enter Range**
**15>/Format,Entry,**

The entries that you want to format are the months in column B, rows 5-11. You also want to move "Date" in B3, so enter

**B3:B11**[RET]

Now the computer responds

**Define Formats: (I,G,E,$,R,L,TR,TL,*,D)**
**18>/Format,Entry,B3:B11**

You want to right justify the text, so type

**TR**[RET]

TR stands for text right. Your screen should now look similar to the one in Figure 6.5.

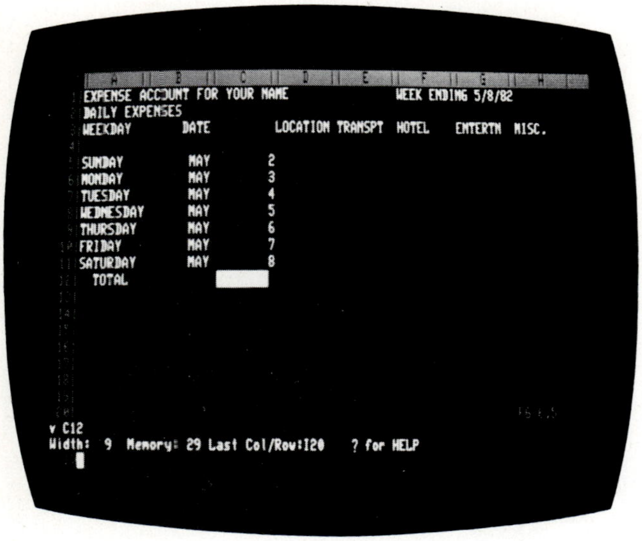


Figure 6.5 Right-justified text

What would you do to left justify the dates? Try this approach; enter

**/FCC**[RET]

which will instruct SuperCalc to FORMAT column C. The numbers should be left-justified in order to be closer to May. To give instructions to left justify, type

**L**[RET]

Your sheet should look like the one in Figure 6.6.

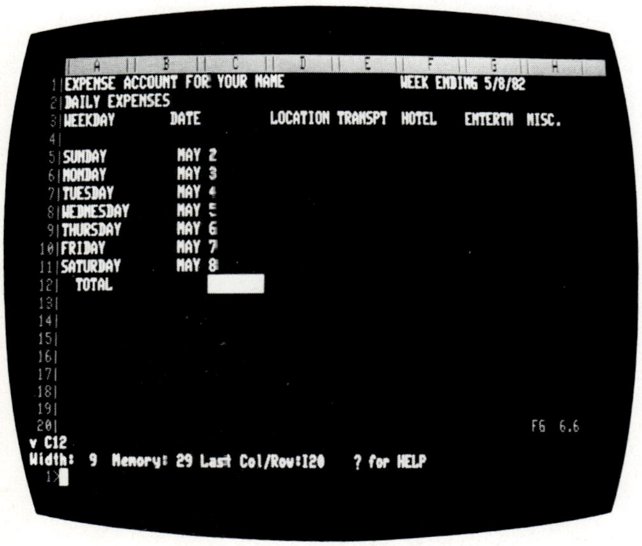


Figure 6.6 Left-justified numbers

## ENTERING INFORMATION

You are now ready to begin entering information into your expense account. Your first entry will be in D5, where you will enter the LOCATION for Sunday, May 2, 1982. On that date, you visited the windy city of Chicago. In fact, you spent the whole week there. Use GO TO to get to D5 by typing

**=D5**[RET]

Then, to enter Chicago in D5, type

**"Chicago**[RET]

REPLICATE the word Chicago for the whole week (make certain your cursor is pointed down). To do this, type

**/R**

In response to **From?**, enter

**D5**[RET]

You want Chicago from D6 to D11 since you were there all week, so in response to **To?**, type

**D6:D11**[RET]

and your screen should look like the one in Figure 6.7.

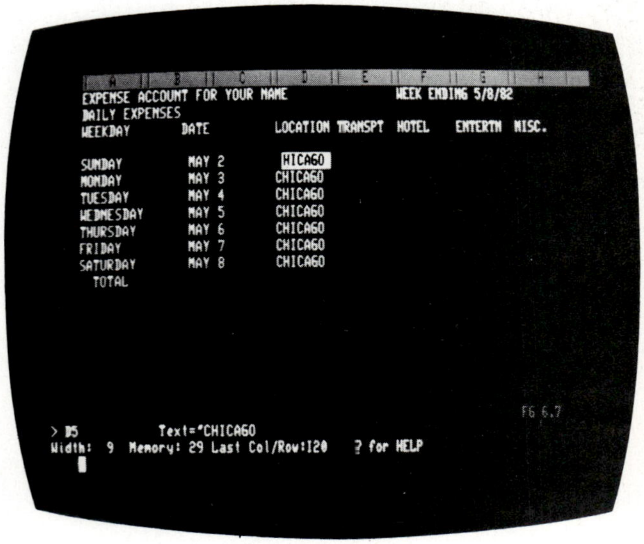


**Figure 6.7** Chicago replicated

Now that you know where you were, let's see how much it cost you to stay there. Move your cursor under HOTEL by using the GO TO command and specifying the cell:

**=F5**[RET]

The first three days you were in Chicago, you stayed at a hotel that cost you $53.14 a night, so type

**53.14**[RET]

REPLICATE this amount into F6 and F7. The command sequence is

**/R**

to replicate, and enter

**F5** RET

to instruct SuperCalc to take information from F5. To put the data into F6:F7, enter

**F6:F7** RET

You moved on Wednesday to a nicer hotel that cost you $72 a night. You stayed there for two nights, so position your cursor at F8 and type

**72.** RET

Now you can either replicate this amount at F8 or type it in. Your display should look like the one in Figure 6.8.

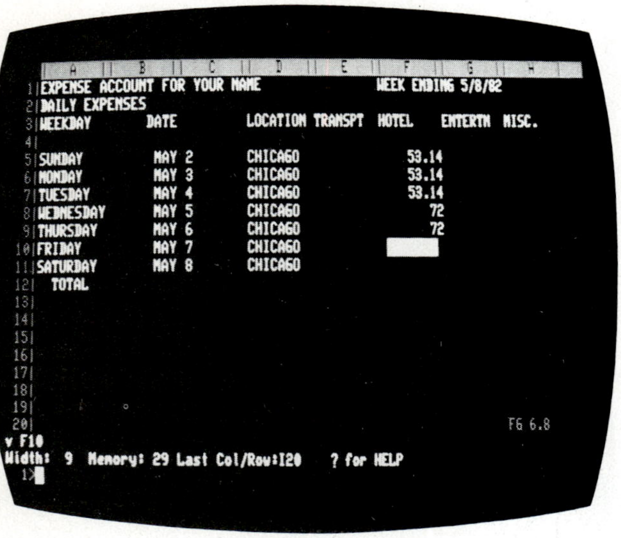


**Figure 6.8** Hotel costs entered

### $ Format and Integer Format

There is a problem. The $72 in F8 lines up under the 14 cents in F7. This makes the expense account hard to read, but you can change it. You can change all of the numbers in the worksheet to a dollars and cents format. FORMAT is a command and must be preceded by a /. To start the FORMAT sequence, type

**/F**

Notice that the prompt line changes to the same display as when you used FORMAT to right and left justify the month and dates. This time, however, you want to change all of the entries on the worksheet. To get a GLOBAL format, enter

**G**

Not only do you want everything formatted, you want it to look like dollars and cents. To do that, use the $. Type

**$** RET

Now all of the numbers, including the dates, are in a dollar and cents format. Your screen should look like the one in Figure 6.9. Since you don't want the dates

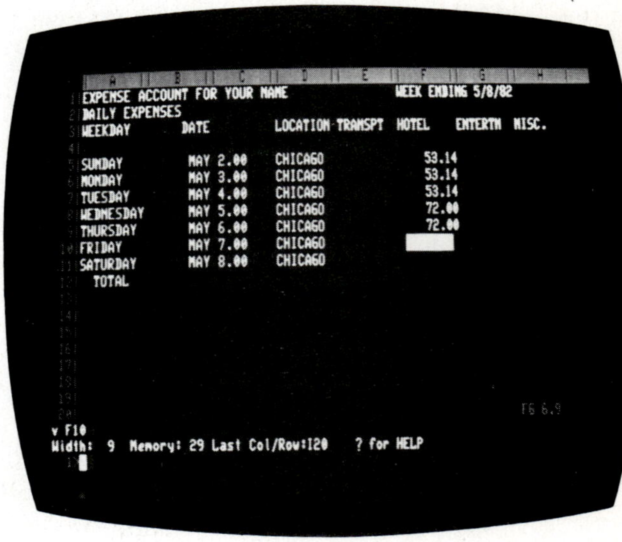


**Figure 6.9** Dollar and cents format

in the dollars and cents format, you can change column C to an integer format (an integer is a whole number). To change the format of numbers in column C type

**/FCC** RET

To get the Integer option, enter

**I** RET

Your display should now look better, like the one in Figure 6.10. The dates should all be in integer format, but the money amounts should have remained in dollars and cents format. The ability to have more than one format on the screen at one time is a valuable feature.

### COPY Command

On Friday, you went back to your first hotel. You will use a new command, COPY, to enter your hotel charges for the last two days. The command for copy is C, but first, GO TO F10 by typing

**=F10** RET

To begin the COPY sequence, enter

**/C**

and you will see the following message:

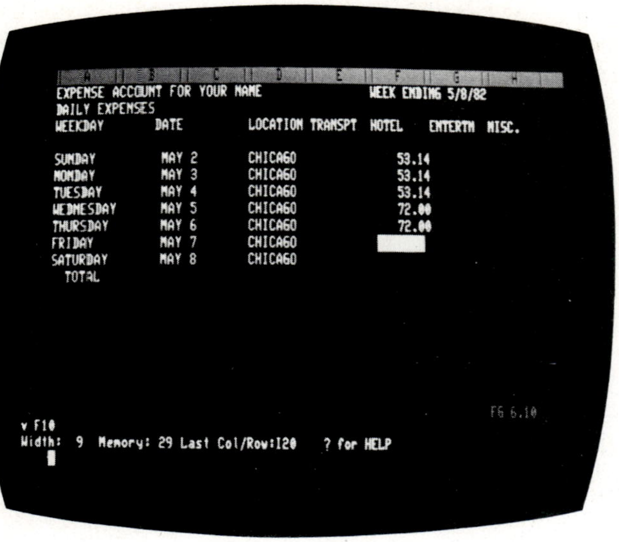


**Figure 6.10** Integer format for dates

**From, (Enter Range)**
**7>/Copy,**

To have the "53.14" price copied from cells F5 and F6 enter

**F5:F6**RET

You may wonder why it was necessary to request information from two cells, especially since the material is the same in both. The reason is that COPY will transfer material to only one cell at a time. In order to get the data into two cells, you must request it from two. When you have entered the line above, the program will respond

**To? (Enter cell), then Return; or "," for Options**
**13>/Copy,F5:F6**RET

Now you will need to designate where you want the information placed. Because you requested data from two cells, you do not have to specify two receiving cells. SuperCalc will automatically put the data in the requested cell (F10) and the cell below it (F11). Type

**F10**RET

and the values in F5 and F6 will be copied into F10 and F11.

You have now been introduced to two very similar commands, COPY and REPLICATE. Although these commands have similar attributes, they do have different uses. The COPY command copies a block of information into a new location starting at a specified cell. The REPLICATE command repeats a block of information into a group of cells. You will better understand how these commands differ as you use them further.

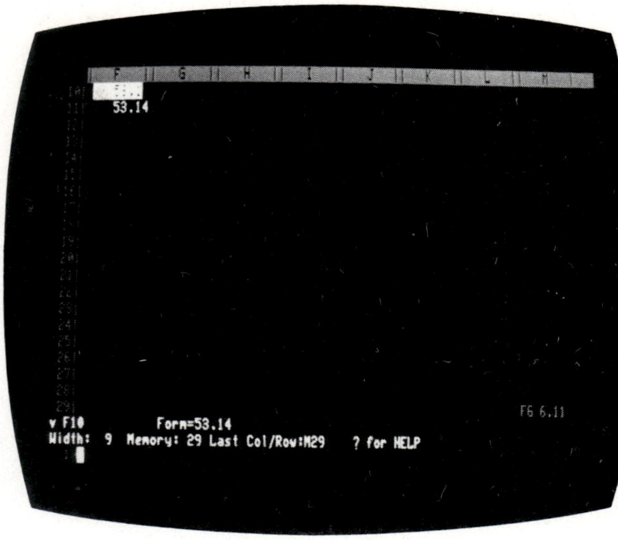


**Figure 6.11** Hotel costs copied

Your screen should now look like the display shown in Figure 6.11. This would be a good time to save your worksheet. To SAVE your work (again called "Expense") on Drive B, type

**/SB:EXPENSE**RET

and the following message will appear

**File already exists: C(hange name), B(ackup), or O(verwrite)?**
**16>/Save,B:EXPENSE**

To get a backup of this worksheet, a B will be entered.

**B**

The next prompt will ask

**A(ll), V(alues), or P(art)?**

You want to save it all, so type

**A**

### SUM Function

Now that you have entered your hotel expenses, let's see how much your hotel bill was in Chicago the week of May 2, 1982. SUM is a built-in function. SuperCalc provides many built-in functions, including SQRT (square root), AVERAGE (arithmetic mean), NPV (net present value), IF conditionals and others that will be discussed in this chapter, in Chapter 8 and in Chapter 10. For SUM, you can specify both ranges and cells. For example, SUM(A8,B9:B12) is equivalent to A8+B9+B10+B11+B12. Position your cursor at F12. To determine the cost of your trip using the SUM function, type

**Sum(F5:F11)**RET

Cell F12 should now display the total 409.70. If your total is not the same check the cells you requested to be summed. Are they exactly as above? If they aren't, just retype the entry. If they are, go back and check each day's hotel cost for an error. Your display should look like the one in Figure 6.12.

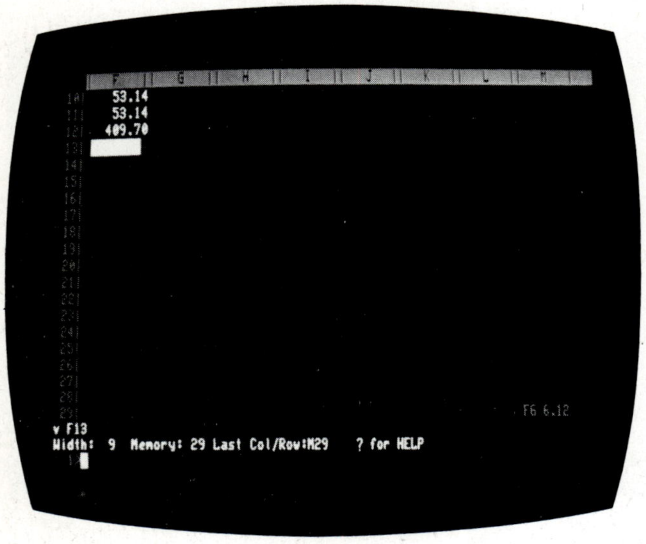


**Figure 6.12** Sum of hotel expenses

You will also want totals in the other expense columns, so let's do that also. You could type in the formula **SUM(F5:F11)** in each of the other columns (substituting E5:E11 for Transportation, G5:G11 for Entertainment, H5:H11 for Misc., and I5:I12 for Total) but that would be somewhat time consuming. Which would be better, REPLICATE or COPY? Remember, with COPY you will specify only the beginning cell and with REPLICATE you will specify a block of cells. Let's use REPLICATE. To replicate the formula for a total you arrived at in F12 in cells E12, G12, H12 and I12, type

**/R**

after which the computer will respond

**From? (Enter Range)**

and you will reply

**F12**[RET]

The prompt line then reads

**To? (Enter Range), then Return; or "," for Options**

You will enter a range by responding:

**E12:I12**[RET]

Your worksheet should now look like the one shown in Figure 6.13.

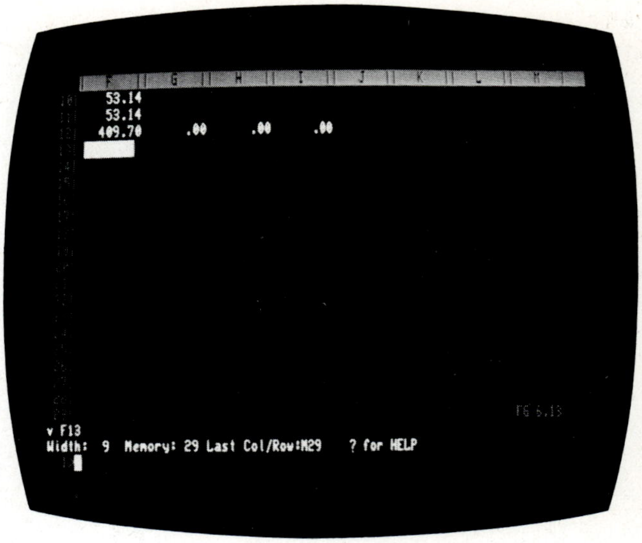


**Figure 6.13** Replicated totals

You may want to use your cursor and scroll over to column I just to make sure the formula was replicated there. As you move the cursor to the right, keep it in row 12 and watch the prompt line to see the different formulas appear. When the program replicated the formulas into cells E12 through I12, it adjusted each entry. In other words, the formula for E12 is SUM(E5:E11), the formula for G12 is SUM(G5:G11) and so on. This is why every total except HOTEL is a 0. When you add numbers into the other columns, the totals will automatically change. As an example, position your cursor at E5 and type

**100**[RET]

The total at E12 will change to 100. You have more entries to make, so let's move on to the next section. The entries for Transportation, Entertainment and Misc. will all be computed on another part of the expense account and transferred to this section. (This would be a good time to SAVE.)

### PARTIAL LOAD and BLANK Commands

The next section of your expense account is called Expense Detail. You will use the same procedure to create it that you used to create the Daily Expense Section. Start by using the COPY command to list the days of the week from A14 to A22. To start, GO TO A5 by typing:

**=A5**[RET]

What you want to do now is give the command to copy the contents of A5 (Sunday) through A11 (Saturday) into the cells starting with A16. To do this, type

**/CA5:A11**[RET]
**A16**[RET]

This instructs SuperCalc to copy the contents of A5:A11 into A16 and those cells below A16. The last cell shown on your worksheet window is A20, so you will not be able to see the words Saturday and Sunday. To see them, use the down arrow to scroll the worksheet so that A22 is visible. Your display should look like the one in Figure 6.14.

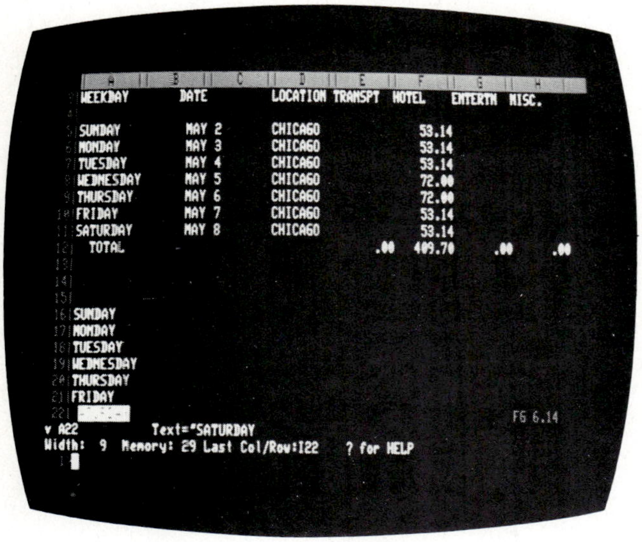


**Figure 6.14** Copied days of the week

There are two other ways that you could have entered the weekdays. You could have used the REPLICATE command or you could have used the PARTIAL LOAD command. Erase the weekdays from the worksheet and reenter them with a PARTIAL LOAD. To erase, use the BLANK command. Type

**/B**

and you will be asked to enter a range. You want to erase the days of the week from A16:A22, so enter

**A16:A22** [RET]

and the entries will be erased. You can BLANK anything from a single cell to the whole worksheet. The next step is to tell SuperCalc that you want to load "Expense" from Drive B. Type

**/LB:EXPENSE** [RET]

and you will be asked

**A(ll) or P(art)?**

You only want to enter the days of the week, so type

**P**

Then it will ask for a range and **From?** You want the information from A5 to A11, so type

**A5:A11** [RET]

Next, it will ask where you want to put the information by asking **To?** You want the information started at A16, so enter

**A16** [RET]

The program will load the days of the week from your saved worksheet starting at A16. (To see A21 and A22, move your cursor down. Notice that as you scroll down to A22, A1 and A2 disappear off the top of the window.) Your display should look like the one in Figure 6.15.

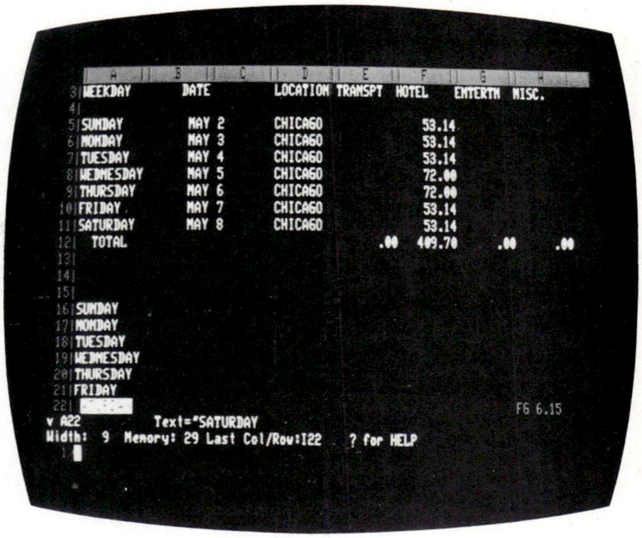


**Figure 6.15** Partial load

The /**L** instructs the computer to load, the **B** determines which drive, **P** indicates a partial load, **A5:A11** says what portion to use, and **A16** gives directions as to where the information should be placed. This command allows you to load parts of one worksheet into another.

Now you can create a header for the next portion of your expense account. This header will start in A14, so GO TO A14 by typing:

**=A14** [RET]

Next, enter the heading starting in A14 by typing:

**"EXPENSE DETAILS** [RET]

You want to GO TO B15, so enter

**=B15** [RET]

Across row 15 you will enter headings for the specifics of your expenses. With the cursor in B15 and pointed to the right, enter

**"TRANSPORT** [RET]
[RET]
**"MISC.** [RET]

TRANSPORT is used here for transportation and the MISC. is used for miscellaneous expenditures. You should have TRANSPORT in B15 and MISC. in D15. You will want two entries each for TRANSPORT and MISC., one to describe the cost and another to enter the amount. Therefore, the next thing to do is to copy the headings into F15, and H15. Do this with the COPY command, and enter

**/CB15** [RET]

This instructs SuperCalc to copy material from B15. In response to **To?**, respond

**F15** [RET]

This tells where you want the material placed. To copy MISC. from D15 to H15, the COPY sequence must be started again. Type in the following and see if you understand each step as it occurs:

**/CD15** [RET]
**H15** [RET]

MISC. should now appear in H15 and your worksheet should look like the one in Figure 6.16.

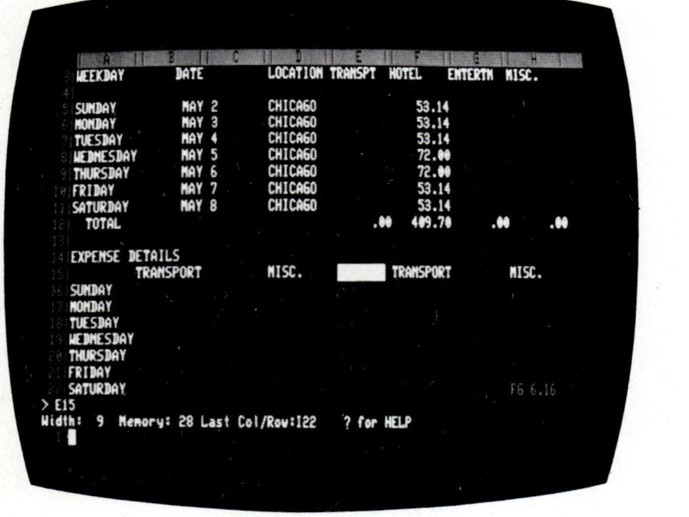


**Figure 6.16** Copied headers

There are subheadings that need to be included under TRANSPORT and MISC. But where can they be placed? Row 15 contains the headings, and rows 16 through 22 have already been designated for reporting daily expenses. You could BLANK rows 16 through 22, enter the subheadings in row 16, and then use the PARTIAL LOAD command again to enter the days in rows 17 through 23.

But there's an easier way to do it, using the INSERT command. To find out how this works, enter

**/I**

and the prompt line will respond

**R(ow) or C(olumn)?**

You want to insert an extra row between rows 15 and 16 to make room for the subheadings, so enter

**R**

Then you will be instructed

**Enter row number**

You should type

**16**

Now there should be an empty row 16 for your subheadings. SuperCalc has moved everything from row 16 down one row. Now, instead of having Saturday in A22, it's in A23. Just to be sure, scroll down and look. Your worksheet should look like the one in Figure 6.17. (When you add rows or columns, SuperCalc generally adjusts any formulas that are affected.)

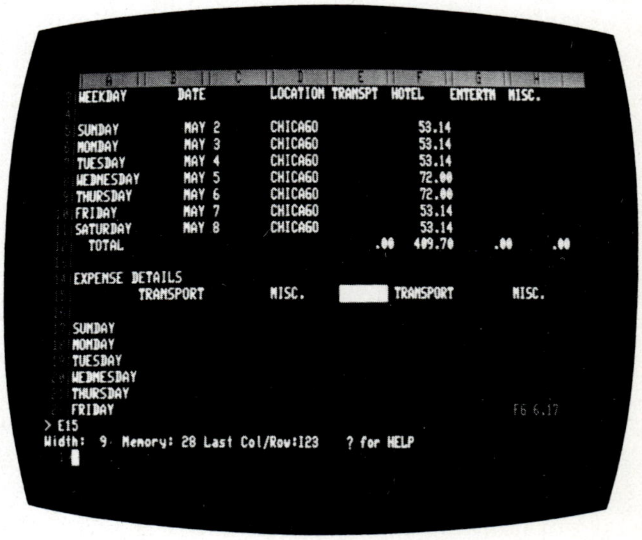


**Figure 6.17** Inserted row

The INSERT command can be used to add a new, empty row or column. However, if you create a new row, anything in row 254, the last one on the sheet, is eliminated. A new column eliminates anything that is in column BK.

Two other SuperCalc commands, MOVE and DELETE, work like INSERT. MOVE can be used to transfer the contents on one entire row or column to another location on the screen. The source row or column is deleted and a new one is created at the destination row or column. DELETE can be used to completely remove a row or column from the worksheet.

Another command, BLANK, will create empty cells in rows or columns, but BLANK does not eliminate the row or column. DELETE not only eliminates the contents of the row or column, it eliminates the location as well. If row 5 is deleted, row 6 is pulled up one row and becomes row 5. Every row below the row deleted also moves up one. If a column is deleted, every column to the right shifts over one location. Your worksheet should not look like the one in Figure 6.17. You are now ready to enter the subheadings under TRANSPORT and MISC. GO TO B16. The titles here are to be AMOUNT (to list each cost) and KEY (to explain what the cost is for). With the cursor in B16 and pointing to the right, enter

**"AMOUNT** [RET]
**"KEY** [RET]

Each of the headings needs a subheading, so you will need to copy AMOUNT into D16, F16 and H16. KEY will have to be copied into E16, G16 and I16. Each cell will have to be copied individually, so to start copying AMOUNT, enter

**/CB16** [RET]
**D16** [RET]
**/CB16** [RET]
**F16** [RET]
**/CB16** [RET]
**H16** [RET]

Once B16 was copied in D16, you could have copied from D16 to F16. It doesn't matter because they all contain the word AMOUNT. For example, to copy KEY:

**/CC16** [RET]
**E16** [RET]
**/CE16** [RET]
**G16** [RET]
**/CG16** [RET]
**I16** [RET]

Your display should now look like the one in Figure 6.18.

### Text Left and Text Right

As you can see, your expenses and their explanation are crowded on top of each other. Why did that happen? Two reasons: first, the cell width is still set at nine spaces and that is too small to accommodate all the letters in some words; and second, text is always left-justified unless you change it. If you were to line up the text to the right side of each cell, then everything would be more readable. Adjusting cell width will be explained later, so for now concentrate on moving the letters to the right side of the

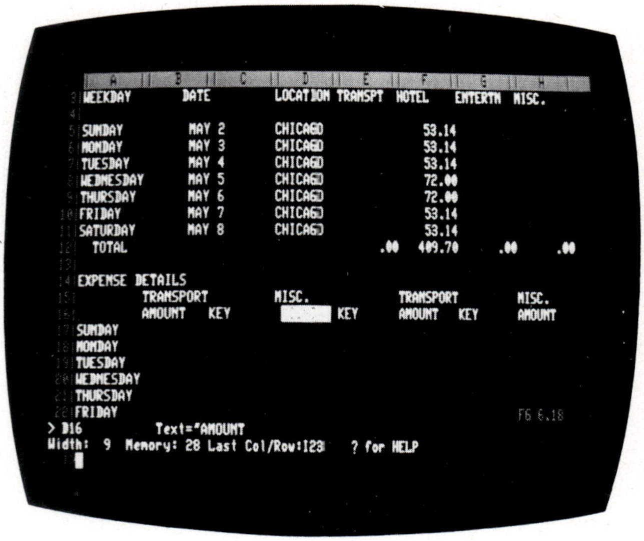


**Figure 6.18** Subheadings

cell. To do that, you must again use the FORMAT command. Enter

**/F**

and the screen will display:

**Enter Level: G(lobal), C(olumn), R(ow), or E(ntry)**

Right now, you want all of the text, or Global formatting, so type

**G**

and watch the screen respond with

**Define Formats: (I,G,E,$,R,L,TR,TL,*,D, column width)**

You want all text moved to the right of the cell (text right), so enter

**TR** [RET]

Your display should now look like the one in Figure 6.19.

First of all, look at the top line (row 1) of your expense account. It doesn't display all of the information you entered. Also, the entries in column A look a little odd. Having the text right-justified seems to be a good idea except for those instances. We can fix column A by formatting just that one column. The sequence to format column A is

**/FCA** [RET]

You want the text in column A moved to the left, or Text Left. Enter

**TL** [RET]

to get a display like the one in Figure 6.20. Notice that part of the information in row 1 reappeared.

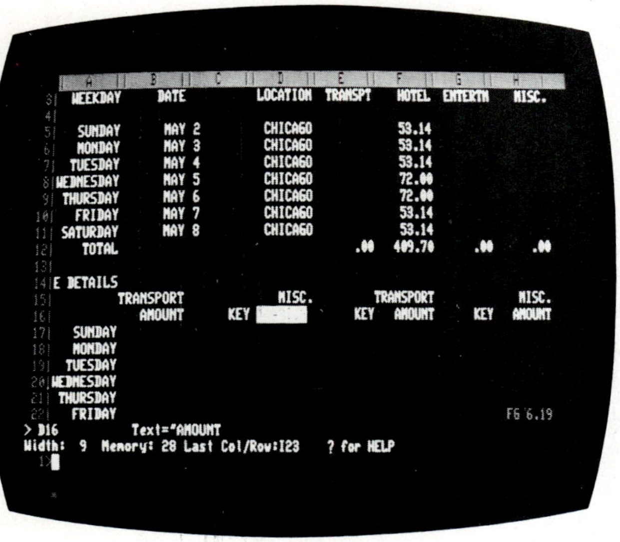


Figure 6.19 Right-justified text

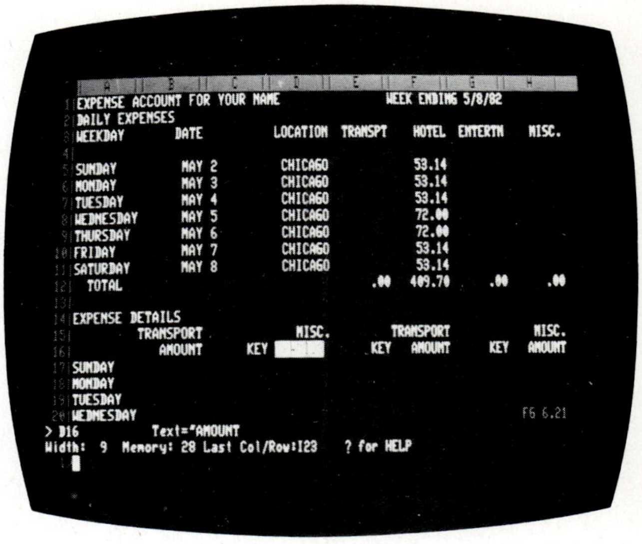


Figure 6.21 Row justification of text

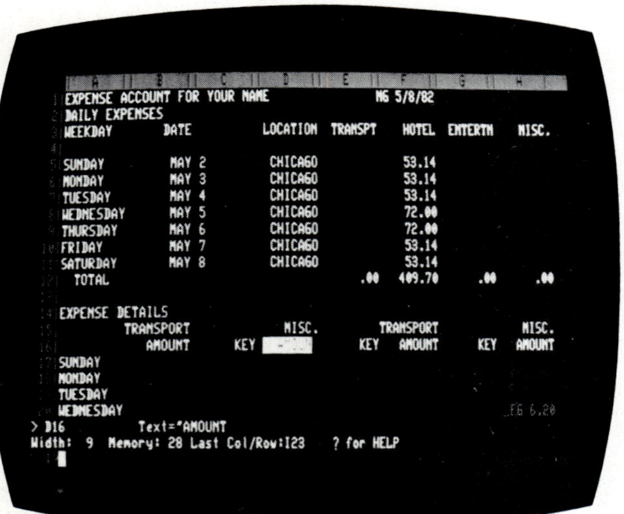


Figure 6.20 Left-justified text

The header, EXPENSE ACCOUNT FOR YOUR NAME, should now be displayed from column A through column D. But what about the rest of row 1? To get the remaining headers, you will want to format row 1 by entering:

**/FR1** RET

To get the information in the headers moved to the left of the cells, type

**TL** RET

SuperCalc added the rest of your information in row 1 so that you should now have a display like the one shown in Figure 6.21.

If you have been working for some time, you may want to stop here and save your work. Please save it on Drive B under the file name of "Expense."

**More Addition**

Now you're ready to put the total TRANSPORT costs in the Daily Expense section of the worksheet. In E5 you will want to enter airfare and taxi costs from the Expense Details Section of the worksheet. That means you need to enter a formula that will take the value of B17 ($441.00 for airfare) and add that to the value of F17 ($22.00 for taxi) and enter the sum into E5 (Sunday transportation cost). That formula is B17+F17. GO TO E5 and enter

**B17+F17** RET

The sum of $463.00 should appear in cell E5. Did the TOTAL in A12 also change? It should now be $463.00, too. Move your cursor back to E5 and look at the status line. It should read

**E5 Form=B17+F17**

Move the cursor and watch the message disappear. Remember that the formula always appears in the status line but that the resulting value is always displayed in the worksheet. Sunday is not the only day for which you will want the transportation costs, however. You will want transportation costs for the rest of the week too. To get the formula in each of the other rows, REPLICATE is the best command to use. Enter

**/RE5** RET

to instruct SuperCalc to replicate the formula in E5. You want the information to go to E6:E11, so type

**E6:E11** RET

Your worksheet should now look like the one in Figure 6.22. Move the cursor down to E7 and look at the status line. It should read

**B19+F19**

Now move the cursor down to E8. The formula should have changed to

**B20+F20**

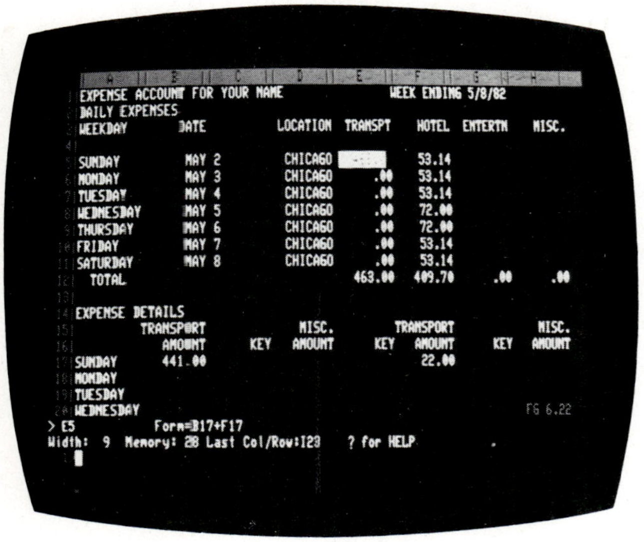


**Figure 6.22** Replicated formulas

What is happening? For each day (row) in the Daily Expenses section, the formula or equation used in column E was changed to take the correct values from the Expense Details section. SuperCalc automatically changed the formulas so that the transportation costs, say for Tuesday, in the Daily Expense section is derived from the Tuesday values in the Expense Details section.

The next step would be to make entries for MISC., but let's work out the formulas first. You want to develop a formula that will allow you to total the two MISC. values from the Expense Details section for each day and transfer that value to the MISC. entry in the Daily Expense section. To do that for Sunday, D17 and H17 must be added together (D17+H17). That's the total for Sunday. To get that total into the Daily Expense section, it must be entered in H5. So, GO TO H5 and enter

**D17+H17** RET

Then replicate this with

**/R** RET **H6:H11** RET

The only change this should have made in your worksheet is that .00 appeared in H5 through H12. (Your worksheet may have moved to the right, if your cursor was pointed to the right, so that column A might have disappeared and column I might now be visible. This movement would be caused by the direction of the cursor, however, and not by entering the formula.)

The Daily Expense portion of your expense account is nearly complete. One other thing to do is total the various entries in the TOTAL cells in column I. Move to I15. (If you GO TO I5, everything to the left and above that cell may scroll off of the screen so that I5 will be in the upper lefthand corner. That may be a little confusing; you might want to use the arrow keys to move the cursor to I15 and not lose so much of the worksheet). To get the total of each day's expenses, you need a formula to total across each category. You could devise such a formula, but it is quicker to use the built-in function, SUM. SUM adds together the values you specify. For example, you want the values from E5 to H5 totaled so that you can see how much was spent on Sunday. You want this entered in the TOTAL column (I). To do this in I5, enter

**SUM(E5:H5)** RET

The total in I5 should be $516.00. Now, you want to know how much you spent each of the other days you were in Chicago. Remember that you used REPLICATE to enter formulas in several cells. Once again, this is the best command to use. Enter

**/R**
**I5** RET
**I6:I11** RET

to start the REPLICATE command. I5 tells the program where to get the information to use, and I6:I11 tells where the information is to be placed. Your worksheet should look like the one in Figure 6.23.

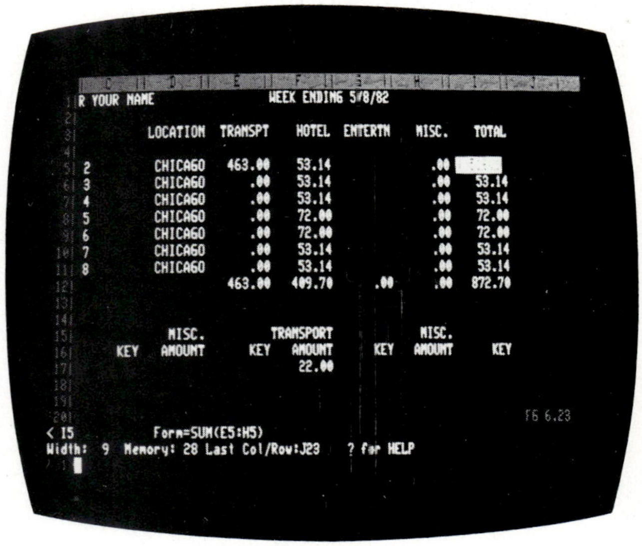


**Figure 6.23** Sum total

At this point your TOTAL column should be essentially the same as the HOTEL column, except for Sunday since you have not yet entered costs in any other day. The display may look a little strange because column A has scrolled off the side of the screen in order to make room for column I. The important thing is that your figures are the same as in the display.

Now you can enter more values in the MISC. and TRANSPORT categories. Place your cursor at B18 and make sure the direction is to the right. On Monday, you rented a car and had several charges for parking. To enter the cost for parking, enter

**9**RET
**"Parking**RET

so that 9.00 shows up in B18 and Parking is in C18 under the heading KEY. You bought $5.00 worth of flowers on Tuesday, so with the cursor in D19 and the position to the right, enter

**5**RET
**"Flowers**RET

The cost should be under MISC. and Flowers should be in E19. By Wednesday, you had driven around so much that you had to put gas in the car. To reflect this as a transport charge, position the cursor over B20 and enter

**16.82**RET
**"Gasoline**RET

Also on Wednesday, you had another parking charge. You already have one transport charge, so use the one in column F. In F20, enter

**9**RET
**"Parking**RET

Your worksheet should now look like the one in Figure 6.24.

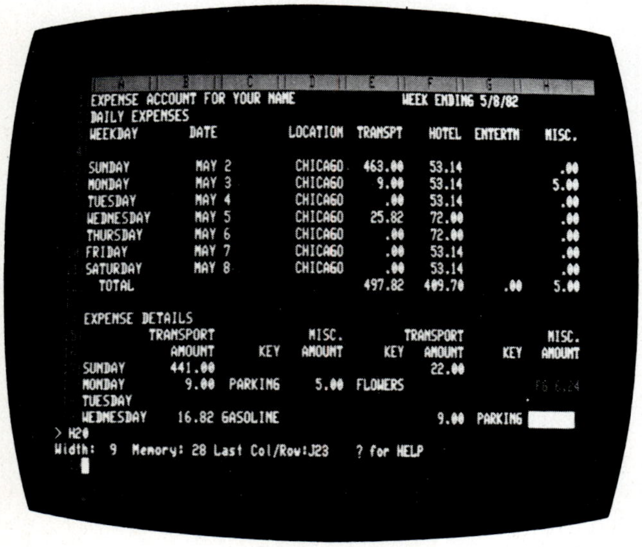


**Figure 6.24** Expense details

**Recalculation**

You may have noticed that each time you enter something into a cell and press RET, the status line displays

**Calculating**

This means that the program is automatically computing the values in columns E and H in the Daily Expenses section. Scroll over to I12 where you can see that the TOTAL expenses have increased to $907.52.

You are now ready to enter your expenses for Thursday. First of all, you paid $12 for parking. Your clothes also finally got back from the cleaners with a bill of $22.37. With the cursor in B21 and the cursor direction to the right, enter the parking charge by entering:

**12**RET
**"Parking**RET

Next, put in the $22.37 for the cleaning by typing:

**22.37**RET
**"Cleaning**RET

Your worksheet should now look like the one in Figure 6.25.

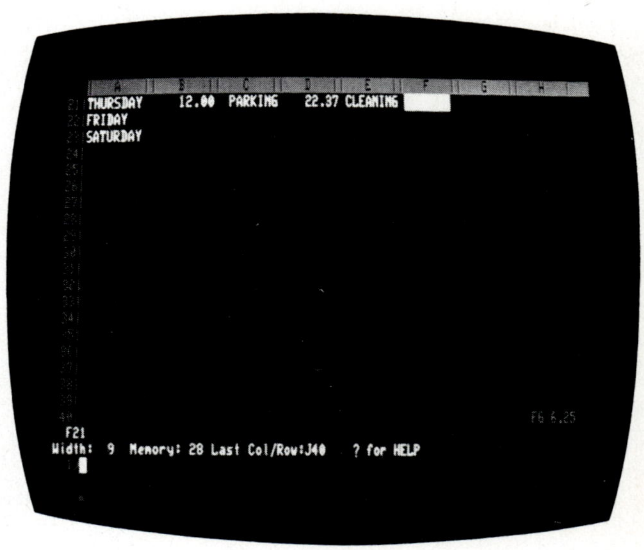


**Figure 6.25** Expenses for Thursday

Even though you stayed in Chicago on Friday and Saturday, you turned the car in on Friday. To enter your car rental expense ($287.19), position the cursor in B22 and enter

**287.19**RET
**"Car Rental**RET

The unusual thing about the appearance of your worksheet now is that row 21 looks like this:

**21 FRIDAY 287.19ar Rental**

Notice that the “C” in Car is hidden. Remember that SuperCalc will display everything in a cell no matter how long it is, *unless* there are numbers or formulas in the adjoining cell. In this case, Car runs into the cell with the car rental amount so that the “C” is omitted. However, if you position the cursor over C21 and look at the status line, the entire message is present. All the information you enter is kept in memory; what is displayed in the worksheet is limited. You can change cell C22 to “Car Rnt and everything will fit in the cell. You could also use FORMAT to make the column wider.

**Window Manipulation**

At last, it’s time to create the Entertainment section of the worksheet. These expenses will be entered in detail in an Entertainment section. The total amount will be entered there and in the Daily Expense section of the worksheet. In order to better compare the two, you will create a *split screen*. A split screen allows you to view two sections of your worksheet together that normally are not displayed together. This example will help explain the “how and why” of split screens. GO TO A13 and type

**/W**

The W command means window and tells the program that you want to change the worksheet window. SuperCalc responds by suggesting different ways in which the window can be displayed. The prompt line now reads

**H(oriz.), V(ert.), C(lear Split), S(ynch.) or U(nsynch.)**

Each option will be used and explained, but for now you want to look at information from the top and bottom of the worksheet. That is called a Horizontal split. To get the horizontal screen, enter

**H**

Your screen should now look like the one in Figure 6.26. Notice that there is a line between rows 12 and 13. Your cursor was at A13 so SuperCalc split the worksheet between rows 12 and 13. You can move the cursor up, down, left or right, within the bottom screen. You will learn how to move from one window to another later in this chapter. The line between rows 12 and 13 is just another border like the one at the top of the worksheet. It is used as a frame of reference.

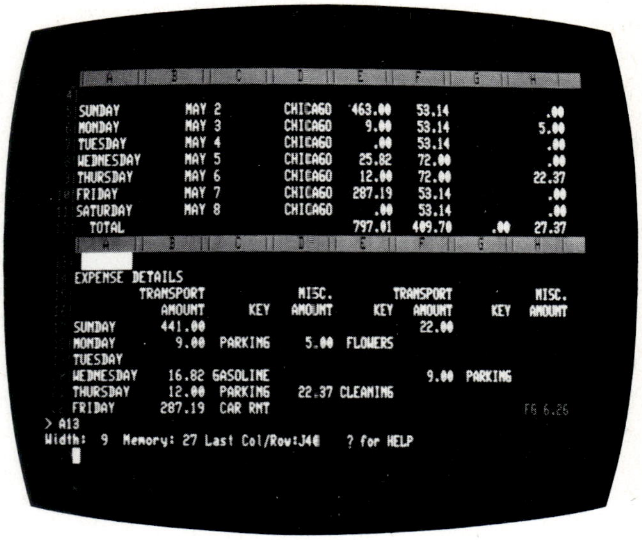

**Figure 6.26** Horizontal window split

Now you can create a heading for Entertainment. GO TO A24 and enter

**“ENTERTAINMENT[RET]**

As a heading under ENTERTAINMENT, you will enter Date, Person, Company, How, Where, Reason and Amount. These will be located in A25, B25, C25, D25, E25, F25 and G25. So, with the cursor in A25 and the direction to the right, enter

**“DATE[RET]**
**“PERSON[RET]**
**“COMPANY[RET]**
**“HOW[RET]**
**“WHERE[RET]**
**“REASON[RET]**
**“AMOUNT[RET]**

Your display should now look like the one shown in Figure 6.27.

Now you can enter information into this section. Position your cursor in A26. Be sure the cursor direction is to the right. On May 3, 1982, you had lunch with Ichabod Crane of Sleepy Hollow at the Mill Restaurant. You discussed pumpkins with him. Lunch cost you $31.40. To enter that information starting in A26, type

**“5/3/82[RET]**
**“ICHABOD[RET]**
**“SLEEPY[RET]**
**“LUNCH[RET]**
**“MILL[RET]**
**“PUMPKINS[RET]**
**31.40[RET]**

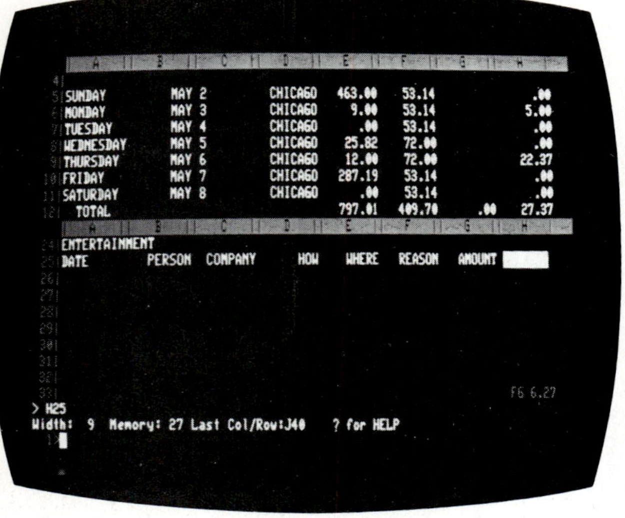


**Figure 6.27** Entertainment headings

How do you enter Ichabod's last name and the rest of the company name? Use the next line for any information that won't fit. One of the nice features of the SuperCalc spreadsheet is that you can put anything anywhere you want. Now, GO TO B27 and enter

"CRANE RET
"HOLLOW RET

Ichabod should now be under the heading of PERSON in B26, and Crane should be in B27. Sleepy should be under the heading of COMPANY in C26 and Hollow in C27.

You want the total for lunch to also appear in the Daily Expenses for Monday. To do that, you can replicate the total in G26 to G6. Simply type

/RG26 RET

to tell the program the information you want replicated, and enter

G6 RET

to say where you want the information placed. You should now have 31.40 in G6 and the TOTAL in that column should also be 31.40.

For dinner on Wednesday, you met Tom Jones of J&S. You arranged the dinner at the "Mart" to establish goodwill with this client. The bill came to $173.22. To enter this information, leave two blank lines between the lunch with Mr. Crane and the dinner. Position the cursor in A29 with the direction to the right and type

"5/5/82 RET
"TOM JONES RET
"J&S RET
"DINNER RET
"MART RET
"GOODWILL RET
173.22 RET

You also want Wednesday's costs in the Daily Expense section. So, as with Mr. Crane, replicate the total in G29 to G8. Enter

/RG29 RET
G8 RET

and you should have 173.22 in G8. Your display should look like the one in Figure 6.28.

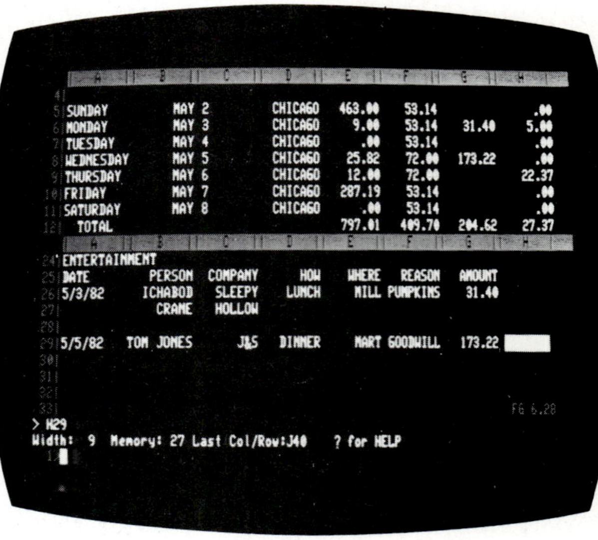


**Figure 6.28** Entertainment formula replicated

In addition, the TOTAL for that column should have changed to 204.62. Remember why? Press the up arrow key until row 12 is the top row in the bottom screen and position the cursor over G12. Look at the status line. That is the formula you entered earlier to tell the program to SUM (add) all the values from G5 to G11.

### Synchronize/Unsynchronize

You have moved around a bit in the lower screen, but when you wanted to look at row 12 you found that you can't move up to the upper screen. Instead, you have to bring the rows down to the lower screen. This is a bit inconvenient. When you set up the split screen, remember the options given by the status line? Those options were

**H(oriz.), V(ert.), C(lear Split), S(ynch.) or U(nsynch.)**

You chose to make a Horizontal split screen.

There is a way to move around within a screen in either the top or bottom portion of the window. The semicolon key (;) is the secret. Use the up arrow key to set up your worksheet so that it displays the same area or window as is shown in Figure 6.28. GO TO A13. Now, press the semicolon key (;). Did you see what happened? The cursor jumped the split screen line. You can now move around in any direction on the top half of the screen by using the arrow keys. What happens when you want to get back to the bottom screen? Use the semicolon key again.

You can move from either window to the other by pressing the semicolon key. Try it a few times. Does there seem to be any kind of pattern to where it appears in a window? GO TO E10 in the upper window. Now, press ;. Where did the cursor go? Press ; again. Where did it go this time? Back to E10. The cursor will return to its last location in either window. Move to F5 and then press ;. It should have gone to its previous location in the bottom window. Now press ; again and watch it go back to F5. But that's only the beginning.

With the cursor in the top part of the window, GO TO K22. The top part of the screen scrolled while the bottom remained in place. This happens because the windows are not synchronized. That is, one window remains still while you scroll in the other. Position the cursor at A1 in the upper window. Again, ask for the WINDOW command by typing:

/W

When the options appear on the status line this time, you want the windows synchronized, so enter

S

Now, move the cursor to K1 by using the right arrow key. See the difference? Both of the windows move together in the same direction. You can GO TO any location from either window and the other window will also move. You may want to try this a few times. When you finish, return your cursor to A1. If you want to move each window separately (unsynchronize them), enter

/WU

Remember that you must first recall the WINDOW command and then choose the Unsynchronize option.

There are two other window commands: V(ertical) and C(lear Split). Clear Split resets the worksheet to a single window format. Vertical allows you to have side by side windows. This feature will be used in the next chapter, but you can experiment with it now. First, clear the split screen. To do that, call up the WINDOW command and select the C option by entering:

/WC

Next, split the screen vertically at column E. GO TO E1, recall the WINDOW command and use the V option. Type

/WV

Your screen should now look like the one in Figure 6.29.

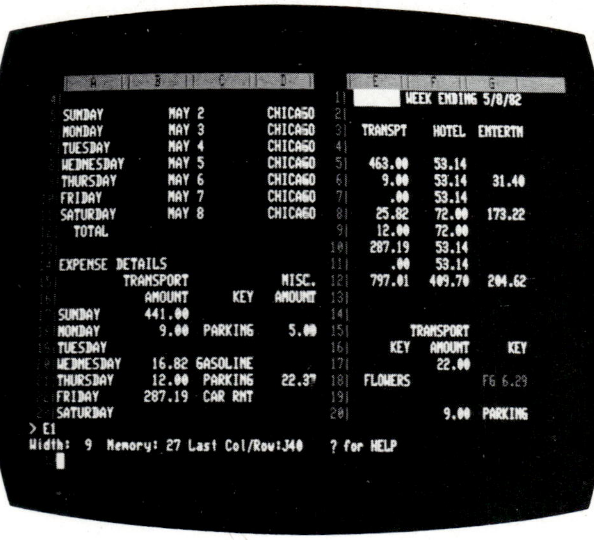


**Figure 6.29** Vertically split screen

This gives you a different perspective, doesn't it? Using this feature, you can enter expenses and watch what happens to the total. You will find many uses for both horizontal and vertical splits.

You will want a horizontal split window to create the Summary section of your expense account, so request a horizontal split. If you enter

/WH

SuperCalc doesn't understand. The status line displays an error message:

**CLEAR Current Split?**

The letters for the options show up on the prompt line. Sorry, you can't just go straight from one type of split to another. It is necessary to first clear whatever type of split might already be in place. Then you can set up another one. In order to get the horizontal split, clear the vertical split by typing:

/WC

Once the screen is in the normal format, and your cursor is at A1, set up the command for the horizontal split by entering:

/WH

It didn't work? Hmmm. Oh, a message on the status line. It reads

**No room (at edge) to display window.**

That means the cursor is on one of the edges of the worksheet and the program can't split at that location. Remember that SuperCalc splits between the row where the cursor is located and the row right above it (or between the column where the cursor is located and the column to the right of it). With the cursor in A1, there is no row above. The same thing would happen if you were at the bottom edge of the worksheet. An error message would appear for a vertical split if you are in the extreme right or left columns. But back to the task at hand. If you position your cursor in A13 again, and enter the sequence for requesting a horizontal split, everything should work out fine this time.

**Expense Account Summary**

You are now ready to create the last section of your expense account. Press the down arrow to set the direction of the cursor and GO TO A37. You want to summarize all of the categories: Travel, Meal, Total, Travel Advance, Credit Card Advance, Total Advance, Due Employee and Due Company. To do that, you will start in A37 and enter

**"SUMMARY**RET
**"TRAVEL EXPENSES**RET
**"MEAL ALLOWANCE**RET
**"TOTAL EXPENSES**RET
**"TRAVEL ADVANCE**RET
**"CREDIT CARD ADVANCE**RET
**"TOTAL ADVANCE**RET
**"DUE EMPLOYEE**RET
**"DUE COMPANY**RET

Ready to enter the expenses? Use the cursor keys to go to D37. You want to copy the value in I12 into D37. Remember that I12 is the SUM of I5 through I11. Now, go back to D37. If you copy this formula into D37, the program will automatically adjust the values. If you try this, however, you will get the SUM of D30 through D36 and this is not what you want. But you do want to copy; you just want to get a little fancy and choose one of the options with COPY. After you have requested the COPY command, and entered the range of I12 and pressed RET, the prompt line responds

**To? (Enter Cell), then Return; or "," for Options**

Press the comma (,) to get the options. Notice that the program has entered D37 on the entry line. It is now the active cell. When using COPY, it is very important to have the cursor at the location where you want the information placed. If your cursor was in a cell other than D37, then another location will be displayed. The prompt line now reads

**N(o Adjust), A(sk for Adjust), V(alues)**

You want only the Values from I12, so enter

**V**

Cell D37 should now have the same value as I12 (1411.33). If your totals in D37 and I12 are not 1411.33, go back and make sure you have entered the values correctly. If the value in D37 is not the same as I12, an error has occurred in the formula. Take a few minutes to check it carefully before going on.

Your TRAVEL expense can be done the same way as the SUMMARY. All you want is to have the TOTAL in the TRANSPORT column (E12) copied to TRAVEL in the SUMMARY (D38). Remember to position the cursor at D38 and then enter

**/CE12**RET
**,V**

The total of $797.01 should now be in D38 and in E12.

**COUNT**

Assume that on this expense account you are given a $20.00 per day meal allowance. To compute this allowance, you need to know how many days you were gone. You could multiply the number of days you were gone (7) by the per diem meal allowance ($20.00) and arrive at an allowance of $140.00. Another way is to let SuperCalc use one of its built-in functions, COUNT, and figure it for you.

COUNT adds all of the non-blank entries in the specified range. That is, it will count all of the entries that have values in them. SuperCalc will COUNT how many entries (days) there are under HOTEL and multiply by the meal allowance ($20.00). For example, if you were to blank F10 (Friday's hotel expense) the value displayed in D39 would be 120.00. If there was a day you were on the road but didn't have a hotel cost, simply enter a 0 for that day. Again, the program counts the number of entries, not the value of each entry. To get this built-in function to work, make sure your cursor is in D39 in enter

**COUNT(F5:F11)*20**RET

You have given instructions to count the number of entries from F5 through F11 and to multiply that number by the per day meal allowance of $20.00. The total of $140.00 should be in cell D39.

**IF**

Now you want to compute TOTAL expenses. That means adding the values of TRAVEL (D38) and MEALS (D39). With your cursor in D40, enter

**D38+D39**RET

The total of $937.01 should now be in D40.

Let's assume that you received a $500.00 travel advance. Also, you charged all of your hotel bill and all of the entertainment expense on your company credit card. This needs to be entered into D41 and D42. With your cursor in D41, type

500

Hotel expenses are in F12 and the entertainment expenses are in G12, so to find the total amount charged on the credit card, the two must be added together. Enter a formula for this calculation in D42 by typing:

F12+G12

The sum of $614.32 should be in D42.

Now, the TOTAL ADVANCE must be computed. The formula for this is D41 (TRAVEL ADVANCE)+D42 (CREDIT CARD ADVANCE). With the cursor in D43, enter

D41+D42

Did you get $1114.32? If not, go over your figures first and make sure they were entered correctly. If there is still an error, check the formulas entered to arrive at total costs. If the total is the same, you are ready to decide who owes whom how much.

To do this, you could subtract the expenses from advances. You could just look at the totals to see if the company owes you money. Or, you can let SuperCalc do it all. Merely subtract D43 (TOTAL ADVANCES) from D40 (TOTAL EXPENSES) and enter the correct amount in D44. That would be fine for this particular trip, because the company owes you money. But what if on the next trip you owe the company money? Then the formula is wrong and you have to recalculate.

To solve this problem, you can use the built-in function, IF. It's probably easier to understand if you enter the formula first and then read the explanation afterward. So, with your cursor in D44, enter

IF(D40>D43,D40−D43,0) RET

What this means is that if the value in D40 (TOTAL EXPENSES) is greater than D43 (TOTAL ADVANCE), then the program will subtract D43 from D40. The result is entered in D44 (DUE EMPLOYEE). If the value of D40 is less than or equal to the value of D43, then the value of D44 (DUE EMPLOYEE) will be zero. You can also compute the value of D44 another way. Enter

If(D40<D43,D43−D40,0)

This means that if D40 (TOTAL EXPENSES) is less than D43 (TOTAL ADVANCE), then D40 will be subtracted from D43. If the value of D40 is, in fact, less than or equal to the value of D43, then the value of D44 (DUE EMPLOYEE) will be zero. So far, the company owes you $297.01. Let's experiment with this a little bit. Change the value in D41 to 1500, and you owe the company $702.99 which is shown in D45. You don't want that, so change D41 back to $500.00. If you are confused about how this works, you might want to read our discussion of conditional expressions in Chapter 10.

**Repeating Text**

About the only things left to do are to make the worksheet fancier and print it out. You can do that by putting in some borders and signature lines. Start by clearing the split windows. Enter

/WC

You can enter a signature line (place for your signature) by using the Repeating Text feature of SuperCalc. The apostrophe is used to start repeating text. Enter the apostrophe and then the character to be repeated. We will use the underline character, but you can use any character your printer can type. With the cursor direction to the right, GO TO A60 and enter

'– RET

Your screen should now have a line across row 60. If you were to scroll across the worksheet, you'd see this line all the way to column BK.

Repeating Text can be applied to the space bar. You can have as many blank spaces as you like. Using the line for your signature as an example, blank out some of the lines. GO TO H60 and enter

'(press the space bar) RET

Did the line disappear from H60 and all other cells to the right? You have erased the line from there to the end of the worksheet. You erased by typing the apostrophe ('), pressing the space bar and pressing RET. This has also formatted the line so that a continuous line (like the one from A60 through G60) can't be put on that row. You can put a dash (–) in each cell, but a line connecting the cells can't be included now.

You can also print your name under the signature line. GO TO A62 and enter

"YOUR NAME RET

Then create a signature line for whoever approves your expense account by using the COPY command. Enter

/CA RET
A67 RET

The entire line has been copied, so you'll need to erase from H67. To do that, place your cursor on H67 and enter

'(press space bar) RET

Now you can put the expense account supervisor's name under the signature line by placing the cursor in A69 and entering:

**Supervisor's Name**RET

And now the expense account worksheet is finished! After all that work, you will probably want to save your worksheet.

## GLOBAL FORMULA

This chapter will end with a discussion on how to adapt the expense account you created to your company's own form. But before that, let's look at how this worksheet can be reused. A reusable worksheet is called a *template.* Before you can create a template, you must first know which cells have formulas in them. GO TO A1 and enter

**/G**

and the prompt line will respond

**F(orm), N(ext), B(order), T(ab), R(ow), C(ol.), M(an.), A(uto)?**

You are going to change the numbers that were derived values on the worksheet back into formulas. To get the formulas, enter

**F**

and the program will automatically display the formulas within the worksheet. Your worksheet should look like the one in Figure 6.30.

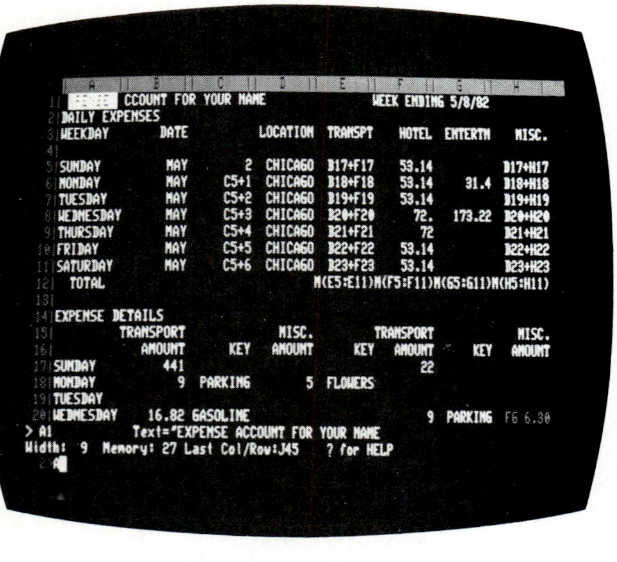


**Figure 6.30** Formulas used in part of the expense account

## CREATING TEMPLATES

When a template is set up, you will be able to enter data into the worksheet easily and conveniently. Start by placing a zero (0) in any cell which will later contain numbers. Enter a quote (") and a blank space in the cells where text will be entered. Take a few minutes to do that now. If you have not saved your worksheet recently, you may want to do it now so that you will have a completed example for reference. You can use the COPY or REPLICATE commands to help blank the cells, but be careful not to disturb the formulas.

## PROTECT

Your next step is to protect all non-entry data. Protect means that the cell or cells cannot be changed or modified. When you use the PROTECT command, you must specify a range or area to be protected. To PROTECT column A, type

**/PA1:A26**RET

Notice that the intensity of protected entries changes immediately (on some terminals) to let you know which areas are protected. You can PROTECT any area of your worksheet. You can also UNPROTECT. If you want to change something in a protected area, use the same procedure as in the PROTECT command (see Chapter 11 for more details). As an example you can unprotect cells A1:A26 by typing

**/UA1:A26**RET

## PRINTING A COPY OF YOUR WORKSHEET

A program that helps you keep track of your expense account wouldn't be all that useful unless you could get a *hardcopy* or printout of the worksheet. The expense account you created begins in the upper lefthand corner of the worksheet at cell A1, extends across the sheet to column I and down the sheet to row 69. When you want to print out your expense account, it will be necessary to tell SuperCalc what part of the worksheet is to be printed. You can do that by using the range A1:I69.

You will also want to get the expense account report printed without the "borders." The borders are the letters across the top and the numbers down the left side. To eliminate borders type

**/GB**

That should remove the borders from your screen display. If you want to put the borders back, all you need to do is give the /GB instruction again. This instruction "toggles" or flips back and forth between the two options. If borders are displayed, it removes them. If they have already been removed, it puts them back in the display.

Now, turn on your printer and be sure it is properly connected to the computer. Put the cursor at A1 and type

**/O**

This is the OUTPUT Command. Super Calc will ask

**D(isplay) or C(ontents) report?**

You want to print what you see on the display so type

**D**

SuperCalc prompts

**Enter Range**

You want A1:I69 so type

**A1:I69**[RET]

SuperCalc then prompts

**Enter Device: P(rinter), S(etup), C(onsole) or D(isk)**

You could select the printer option and begin printing the worksheet now, but it is a good idea to select the C(onsole) option first. That will send the material to the video display rather than to the printer. You can then look at it and spot any problems before the printer is used. Type

**C**

The expense account report will appear on the screen as it would be printed out on the printer, with one exception. (Press the [RET] key or space bar to see each section of the report.) Since the video display is capable of showing only 24 lines of 80 characters at once, it will not show the TOTAL column with the rest of the first part of the report. A standard 8½-inch by 11-inch sheet of paper has room for 66 lines; it can accommodate the full width of the expense account report, including the TOTAL column. (If you have already used the printer and have modified the Setup values, reset then to their default values now. See Chapter 5 or the Reference Section for details.) There is one problem if you are using standard-sized paper. The expense account has 69 lines in it while the standard sheet accommodates only 66. However, there is a simple solution to that problem. Rows 47 through 61 are simply spacers; there is nothing in them. You can use the DELETE command to remove some of them and, if the expense report is single-spaced, make it fit on one page. Type

**/D**

SuperCalc will prompt

**R(ow), C(olumn) or F(ile)?**

This command enables you to remove an entire row or rows, a column or columns, or a complete file which has been stored on a diskette. You want to remove some rows, so type

**R**

SuperCalc then prompts for the row to be deleted. Type

**48**[RET]

SuperCalc then removes row 48 and moves all the rows below it up one row. You will need to repeat this command several times (e.g., /DR48) until your signature line is in row 50. Now the expense report is short enough to fit on one page. Remove the borders with the /GB command again (if you have borders at this point) and you are ready to print. Type

**/ODA1:I59**[RET]

Now be sure your printer is set up, the paper is in place, and everything is connected. Then type

**P**

If something is amiss, you can halt the printing process by holding down the [CTL] key and pressing the **Z** key. If, on the other hand, everything is running smoothly, you should have a printout. After seeing what the printout looks like, you may want to make some adjustments to make it look nicer. That is not difficult. Again, see Chapter 4 and the Reference Section for details on the OUTPUT instruction.

Finally, save your template under a name other than "Expense" because that is the name you've used for examples. "Account" might be a good name.

## SUMMARY

Look at everything you've accomplished. Can you briefly explain how each command is used? The number to the left of each command indicates the page on which it is discussed.

| | |
|---|---|
| BLANK | 41 |
| COPY | 38 |
| DELETE | 42, 53 |
| FORMAT | 36, 38, 43 |
| GLOBAL | 38, 52 |
| INSERT | 42 |
| LOAD | 41 |
| OUTPUT | 52-53 |
| PROTECT | 52 |
| REPLICATE | 35 |
| SAVE | 36, 39 |
| UNPROTECT | 52 |
| WINDOW | 47 |

If you have mastered these commands, you have most of the SuperCalc commands at your fingertips. If you are unclear about the use of any of these, go back and review them. The rest of the SuperCalc commands will be discussed in the next chapter, "Financial Forecasting."

# Chapter 7

# Financial Forecasting

This chapter presents many of the useful features of SuperCalc which have not yet been explained and illustrated. You will learn about SuperCalc by looking at the unique area of financial forecasting. You will examine what it is and why it is important. In addition, you will learn how to develop parameters that make financial forecasting more meaningful. As an introduction, you will use two examples taken from your systems diskette, Balance Sheet which is called BALANCE and a breakeven analysis called BRKEVN. Both are on the diskette that contains SuperCalc. Since forecasting is quite complex, we'll start with the Balance example and then make a few changes in it. Then you will learn how to answer some "what if" type questions using the Breakeven example. To get a feel for how all this fits together, you will then be introduced to worksheet design. Finally, you will learn some additional built-in functions that are extremely useful in forecasting.

To get started, load the Balance worksheet from your diskette. Remember that the command LOAD is entered by typing the letter L and then the file name. When asked if you want A(ll) or P(art) of the worksheet, respond "A." The sequence for this procedure is

**/LBALANCE**RET
**A**

Now that Balance has been loaded, take a look at it to see what's there. It's a good idea to "get the lay of the land" any time you load an unfamiliar sheet, just to have a general knowledge of what's there. For example, how big is this worksheet? Move your cursor to the right until you find the last column with information in it. The last column is N. Now move the cursor down and find which row contains the last piece of information. It's row 25. What else can you find out about this worksheet?

### TITLE LOCK

Use the arrow keys to scroll across the worksheet. Notice how the various headings appear and disappear as you move around the screen. There is a way to move the cells without moving the titles. It is called TITLE LOCK. To see how this works, GO TO A4 and "set" the titles in column A by using the command symbol (/) and the command letter for TITLE LOCK (T). To do that, enter

**/T**

The prompt line will respond with the TITLE LOCK options:

**H(oriz.), V(ert.), B(oth) or C(lear)**

You may have the titles locked in rows (horizontal), in columns (vertical), or in both directions. The C(lear) option erases the TITLE LOCK command. For now, ask for a vertical lock by entering:

**V**

Now press the right arrow several times and watch as the months scroll across the screen and column A remains in place. In fact, if you scroll far enough, column N will be displayed next to column A. Now try to move the cursor to the left into column A. It won't go. The only way you can enter a row or column that has a TITLE LOCK is to use the GO TO command.

TITLE LOCK lets you look at the figures in many rows or columns without scrolling your descriptive headings for those rows or columns off the screen. When you set TITLE LOCK, it is only necessary to have the cursor in a cell of the row or column you want to TITLE LOCK. If you "lock" while the cursor is in column C, however, SuperCalc will lock everything from C back to the left. Thus, columns A, B and C will be locked.

There will be some instances where you will want to lock the titles in a horizontal direction, too. That is, you may have descriptive headings across the top of the sheet that should stay in place as you scroll. To do that you must first clear any vertical lock already in place. Do that by recalling the TITLE LOCK command, and pressing C:

**/TC**

SuperCalc will automatically redefine the screen so that all locks are removed. You can now enter any column or row using the arrow keys. Be sure the cursor is somewhere in row 4 since you want to lock rows 1, 2, 3, and 4. To set the horizontal lock, use the TITLE LOCK command, but this time press the H:

**/TH**

Notice that you are now unable to move the cursor into any of the month names. If you scroll down the worksheet, the headings at the top of the sheet stay in place. Clear the TITLE LOCK with

**/TC**

## GLOBAL FORMULAS AND PROTECT COMMANDS

With the TITLE LOCK cleared, look at the format of the worksheet. Position the cursor at B3 and notice that the status line displays

**P Text="Jan**

What does that tell you? First of all, the **P** tells you that the cell is protected. All of the titles in this row and in column A are half intensity (if your terminal supports more than one intensity) so that you will know which cells are protected. Remember from Chapter 8 that you cannot alter the data in a protected cell.

What formulas are there on the worksheet? To find out, use the GLOBAL command with the Formula option. Type

**/GF**

Your worksheet should look like Figure 7.1. You will see that most of the entries are now formulas. Notice that the entries for the months of February through December are either formulas that depend on prior months or constants repeated from the January column (constants are values that remain the same). The Totals column is made up exclusively of formulas.

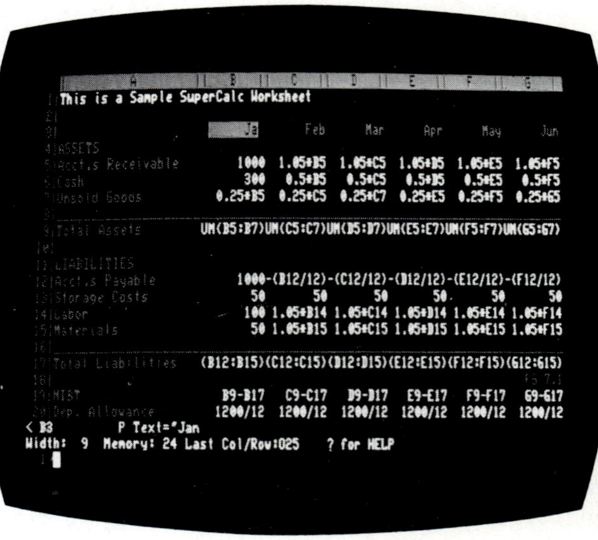


**Figure 7.1** Global formulas

This worksheet is a simple projection that depends on the figures for January. It points up a key element of financial forecasting: all forecasts involve a few primary assumptions extended over a period of time. You can have a very sophisticated forecast that depends only on five or six assumptions.

To change the worksheet back to numbers, use the GLOBAL command and the Formula option again. The Formula option displays formulas but it also "turns off" the option. Enter

**/GF**

Try changing some of the values and notice what effect it has on the rest of the values. For instance, GO

TO B13 and change the Storage Cost from $50.00 to $200.00. To do this, at B13 enter

**200** RET

Only the Total Liabilities in B17 changes. Everything else remains the same. But, if you change the Accounts Receivable in B5 from $1000.00 to $20,000.00, watch how everything outside of the Total Assets category changes! Experiment with the worksheet to get an idea of which changes cause impact and which don't. One of the real values of SuperCalc is that it can help you determine what is important and what isn't. When you have finished with the worksheet you can destroy it with the ZAP command and load in the program for breakeven analysis (called BRKEVN) from your diskette. To use ZAP, enter

**/Z**

and when the entry line asks

**/Zap–ENTIRE–Worksheet?**

respond

**Y**

and the whole thing will go away. Follow the same procedure as before to load the Breakeven Analysis worksheet. When asked for the file name, remember that the name is spelled "BRKEVN." Also, load in "All" of the worksheet.

## WHAT IF

Once you have determined what's important, you are ready to start asking some "what if" questions. As an example of how this is done, look at the Breakeven Analysis sheet. The idea of a breakeven sheet is actually a simple one. When you market a product, there are two types of costs. There are fixed costs, such as development and overhead, and there are variable costs associated with manufacturing the product, such as parts and labor. When you sell the product, you want to price it in such a way that you recover both your fixed and variable costs and make a profit. The breakeven point is the point at which you change from a loss to a profit.

Now look at how the worksheet is constructed. Set the values to formulas by requesting a GLOBAL and Formula display. Do this by entering:

**/GF**

Take a look at column C, Units Sold. Cell C2 has the value of B18, which is the Quantity Increment (100). Cell C3 is C2 plus the Quantity Increment. Cell C4 is C3 plus the Quantity Increment, and so on down the column. The formula for each value consists of the value of the cell directly above, plus the increment.

Next, look at column D, Profit and Loss. These are long formulas, but they do not contain any complicated math. They are just long formulas made up of simple math calculations. Let's start with D2. The formula is

**C2*B3*(.01*(100−B19))−(B9+(B16*C2))**

As you go down the column, you will see that other formulas also look like typographical errors. In D3, the formula is the same. In D4, C3 is replaced with C4. This pattern continues throughout the column. So the formula in D2 starts out with Units (C2) multiplied by Retail Price (B3). The .01 multiplied by (100−B19) subtracts the Discount Rate from 100 and makes the result a percentage. If the value of B19 is 40, then .01(100−B19) equals 60 or 60%. In other words, this expression is the percentage of the Retail Price that you get to keep. It is your wholesale price. What about (B9+(B16*C2))? Cell B9 is the sum of the Fixed Costs. Cell B16 is the Total Variable Costs multiplied by C2 (Units Sold). The formula in D2 is C2 (Units Sold) multiplied by B3 (Retail Price) minus B19 (Costs). When you understand the formulas, change the display back to numbers by using the GLOBAL command with the Formula option by entering:

**/GF**

### Global Command with the Manual Option

Before we work through an example, there is a new option to the GLOBAL command that allows you to enter data into your worksheet rapidly. Normally, as you enter date, the program recalculates all formulas and displays the new totals. When you use the GLOBAL command with the Manual option, the recalculation is done only when *you* want it to be done. This is especially helpful when you have a large worksheet or when you have a lot of data to enter. You don't need to wait for the program to recalculate after each entry. It also helps you keep track of *iterative* calculations (iterative calculations are those formulas that reference the value of their own cell and perform calculations).

To try out this new option, change the Retail Price in B3, the Discount Rate in B19, and the Quantity Increment in B18. To start this process, first choose the GLOBAL command and the Manual option by entering:

**/GM**

Just by looking at the screen, you can't tell that you have entered the Manual option. The display looks the same as before. Change the value of Retail Price in B3 to 19.95, the Discount Rate in B19 to 40, and the Quantity Increment in B18 to 400.

You can now use another feature of SuperCalc called *auto-advance*. Up to now when you entered data and pressed the RET key, the cursor would jump to the next cell. The direction of the jump is determined by the arrow shown on the status line. You can stop the auto-advance feature by typing:

**/GN**

The Next option of the GLOBAL command (selected by typing N) toggles between auto-advance and no auto-advance. If you type /GN when the system is using auto-advance, that feature is turned off. If it is off and you type /GN, it is turned on. Turn the auto-advance off before proceeding.

Next, you want to GO TO B6 and change the Development Costs to $4000.00. After doing that, press the down arrow key once and enter another GLOBAL/Next instruction by typing:

**/GN**

You should now be at cell B7 where you can change the value to 10000. When you enter 10000 and press RET, the cursor will jump down to B8. While in B8, change the value to 2200, then enter the following changes in B12 through B15:

**C=Y**
**.5**RET
**.08**RET
**.02**RET
**.01**RET

Your display should look like Figure 7.2. Note that the other cells on the worksheet do not change even though you have entered new values. To get the

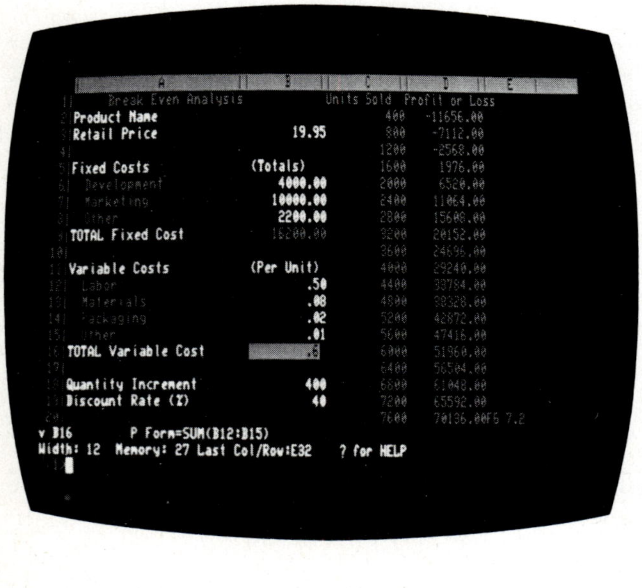


**Figure 7.2** Global manual

values computed, type the exclamation mark (!). As soon as you enter

**!**

you will be able to see the breakeven point. The ! tells the program you want it to calculate the formulas. It will only do that when you enter the !, unless you tell SuperCalc you no longer want to use the manual recalculation option. You can return to automatic recalculation at this point by using GLOBAL and A (for automatic). Enter

**/GA**

## LOOKUP FUNCTION

One of the major variables in this example is Discount, the value entered in cell B19. What effect will different Quantity Discounts have on the breakeven point? You could enter a variety of Quantities and test them against Discounts, but there is a less tedious way.

You can start this by constructing a table of possible Quantities. GO TO cell F1 and enter the header "QUANTITY TABLE" in F1. Here are the commands for the instructions described above:

**C=Y**
**=F1**RET
**"QUANTITY TABLE**RET

If the cursor is not in cell F2, move it to that cell. If the auto-advance option is not on, use the GLOBAL, Next sequence (/GN) to turn it on. Also, be sure the direction of auto-advance is down. Now press the RET key. Your cursor should be in F3. If it stayed in F2, your automatic advance is out of sequence. (Typing /GN once sets the cursor *not* to move after a RET and typing it again sets it *to* move to the next cell after a RET. Type /GN again and it should be fixed.)

With your cursor in F3, the automatic advance turned on, and the direction down, enter

**25**RET
**50**RET
**75**RET
**100**RET
**200**RET
**500**RET
**1000**RET
**2500**RET
**5000**RET
**7500**RET
**10000**RET

Your display should now look like Figure 7.3. Now, start a new column for entering Discounts in G2 by entering:

**/G2**RET

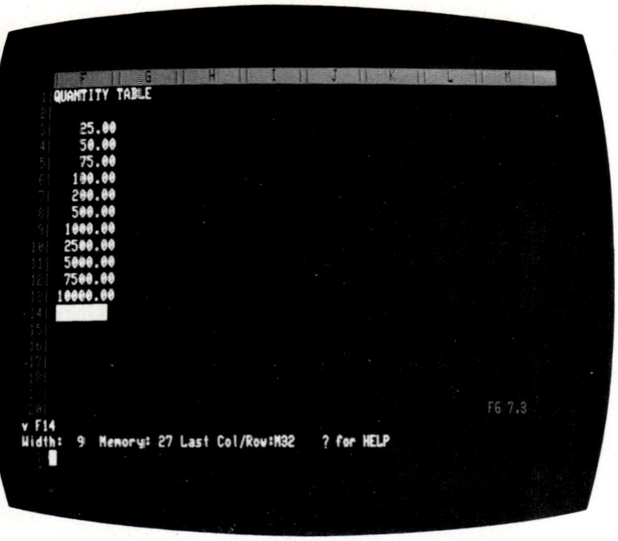


**Figure 7.3** Quantities table

and then typing:

**10**[RET]

Now place the formula G2+5 in cell G3:

**G2+5**[RET]

With the cursor in G4, use the REPLICATE command to place the formula in G3 in G4 through G13. Enter

**/RG3**[RET]
**G4:G13**[RET]

Column G should contain a list of discounts which reflect the relationship between the quantity ordered and the wholesale price. For example, if a customer orders 75 units, the discount off the retail price will be 25%. If 7500 units are ordered, the discount will be 60%.

You are now ready to learn another SuperCalc function, LOOKUP. First, however, you need to set up the display so that you can see columns B through G. To do that, GO TO B11. You actually want to work in B19, so use the down arrow key to arrive at B19.

Now that you're all set, what is the LOOKUP function? LOOKUP is a fairly complex but very useful function. Here is the general format:

**LOOKUP (Search Value, Column or Row Range)**

LOOKUP searches the range specified in the last part of the function until it finds the value that is less than or equal to the Search Value. For example, suppose you have the values below in cells R1 through R6 and S1 through S6:

| Row | Column R | Column S |
|---|---|---|
| 1 | 10 | 50 |
| 2 | 20 | 100 |
| 3 | 30 | 150 |
| 4 | 40 | 200 |
| 5 | 50 | 250 |
| 6 | 60 | 300 |

If you put LOOKUP(23,R1:R6) in cell R21, the value of that cell will be determined by what SuperCalc finds in rows 1 through 6 of columns R and S. First, it will look down column R until it finds the highest number that is less than or equal to the search value. In the example, the search value is 23. Thus, it will select 20 as the largest value that is not greater than 23. Here is where LOOKUP gets a little complex. Instead of putting the number 20 in cell R21, it looks in the cell just to the right of the one containing 20. That is cell S2. It contains the value 100, and that is what SuperCalc puts in cell R21. If our search value were 65, it would match on cell R6 and put the number 300 in R21. If the search value were 49, it would match on cell R4 and put the number 200 in cell R21.

Two things should be remembered about LOOKUP. First, it assumes that the lookup table (R1:R6 in the example) is arranged in ascending order. That is, the lowest numbers in the table come first, larger ones come later. Second, you can use LOOKUP on a row range as well. When used with rows, it gets the value in the cell just below the target cell rather than the cell to the right.

To see how it works in the Breakeven worksheet, be sure the cursor is in B19 and type

**LOOKUP(B18,F2:F13)**[RET]

The LOOKUP function searches for the last value in the range of F2:F13 that is equal to or less than B18. It then returns the value in the adjacent column to the right. For example, if you change the value in B18 to 10, then B19 (Discount) will change to 10. Why? Because the LOOKUP function goes to column F to find the value equal to or less than B18 (10). Finding the value of 10, it then moves to the same row in column G and puts that value of G (10) in B19. If you change B18 to 1000, SuperCalc will search column F for a value equal to or less than 1000. When it encounters 1000, it goes across to column G, finds a value of 45, and returns 45 to B19. What happens if you change B19 to 999? The value changes to 40 because 999 is less than 1000. If you experiment with this a bit, you see that the breakeven point is between 1200 and 1500 units, depending on the discount.

You can use the LOOKUP function to establish other relationships on the worksheet, too. This is a good function to use any time you want to evaluate a group of variables. It lets you change one key variable in one cell and have SuperCalc do the work of looking up the effect of that one change and doing all the recalculating required to judge the effect of that change.

If you add different numbers into this worksheet, you may notice that increases in Fixed Costs mean it will take a little longer to break even, but your long term profits are not altered that much. On the other hand, if the variable costs increase, profits drop even over the long term. You could experiment with the quantity discount and retail price variables to find the relationship that best meets the needs of your company and the marketplace.

Like the other examples in this chapter, this worksheet is realistic, but simplified. You can use it as it is, though, to get a general idea of product pricing policy. You can also use it as an example of short term forecasting that considers actual marketing costs, discounts and price changes.

There are some other ways you might experiment with this worksheet. For instance, you might put changes at intervals in the worksheet. You could have the numbers in the worksheet represent the costs for a six-month interval of production. You could test the number of units produced using the LOOKUP function. Based on that test, you could specify adjustment factors for prices and costs. Then you could multiply your price and cost information by the adjustment factors and refer to the adjustment factors in other formulas. The point is that this worksheet is an excellent experimental tool. By using it, you will gain some valuable experience in worksheet manipulation and become more efficient in using SuperCalc.

## WORKSHEET DESIGN

Like any other complex managerial tool, SuperCalc takes some advance planning to be most useful. Although it is tempting to just sit down and start entering numbers into a worksheet, it is far more effective to set out a plan for developing the worksheet before you begin. Worksheet design consists of asking yourself four questions:

1. What do I want to do?
2. What are the parameters?
3. What are the components of the worksheet (titles, etc.)
4. What assumptions will be made?

Let's work through a simulated worksheet design. The answer to question one (What do I want to do?) is that you want to analyze cash flow generated from selling land over a ten month period. You are going to assume that you will sell one piece of property a month. You will also ask a whole group of "what if" questions. For instance, what if the prime rate is different from what you project, and what if the property fails to sell when you project it will?

In answer to the second question (What are the parameters?), the parameters of your worksheet are as follows: you have ten pieces of property that have the following values:

1. $125,000
2. $275,000
3. $160,000
4. $283,000
5. $365,000
6. $425,000
7. $1,673,000
8. $518,000
9. $227,000
10. $351,000

All of these properties are mortgaged at 65% of their value and you expect to sell them in the order listed for full value. The interest rate is prime plus 2% and you have to pay a sales commission on all land sold. The sales commissions are based on the sales during the particular month that they occur. The sales commission on the first $100,000 is 6%; on the next $100,000, 5%; and on anything above $200,000, 4%.

Now that you know the parameters, you are ready to look at the elements of the worksheet (question 3). To determine the cash flow, you must know two things: what is the cash brought in for each month and how much cash goes out? The cash brought in consists of Sales. The cash out consists of Commissions, Mortgage, Payoff and Interest. In order to get a firm handle on what these elements are, you need to ask a series of questions: what sold this month, how much was paid out in commissions, how much mortgage is remaining, and how much interest will be paid?

Now you are ready to answer the crucial fourth question: what assumptions will I make? Since all forecasting involves some assumptions, this is perhaps the most important question to ask. In this worksheet, let's assume that whenever you sell a piece of property the cash is delivered on the last day of the month and that the sales commission is deducted from it. That means your interest payment covers the entire month. It also means that you can derive the interest payment for February by subtracting January sales from the January mortgage, multiply that mortgage by the interest rate and come up with the interest at that point. Also in

January, you can multiply sales times the commission rate tc see how much net cash you have left over, and you have to compute your mortgage payment. Now you are ready to design the worksheet.

One of the easiest ways to design a worksheet is to lay out exactly what you are going to do on a piece of paper. Our layout for this example is in Figure 7.4. First, we listed the titles across the top of the layout: Month, Mortgage, Sales, Payoff, Interest, Commission, Net Cash and Total Cash. Then we put the months down the side.

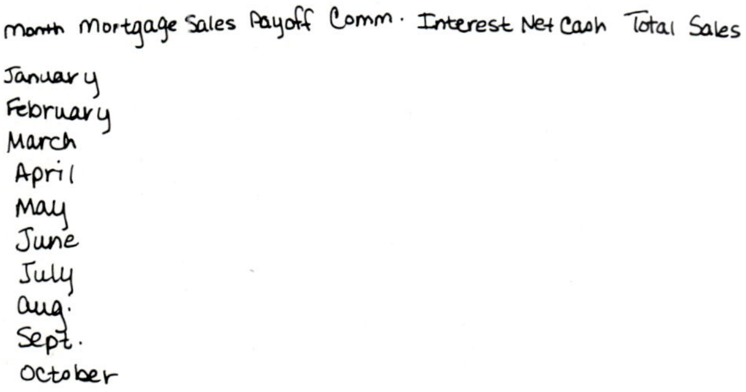


**Figure 7.4** Paper and pencil design

Start wih a clean worksheet. You can either ZAP the breakeven analysis sheet or use the blank worksheet that comes up when you load SuperCalc. At A1, type

**"CASH SALES FORECAST[RET]**

Then, GO TO A2 and begin entering the headings across the top:

**"MONTH[RET]**
**"MORTGAGE[RET]**
**"SALES[RET]**
**"PAYOFF[RET]**
**"COMM.[RET]**
**"INTEREST[RET]**
**"NET CASH[RET]**
**"TOT.CASH[RET]**

GO TO A3 and enter down the page:

**"JANUARY[RET]**
**"FEBRUARY[RET]**
**"MARCH[RET]**
**"APRIL[RET]**
**"MAY[RET]**
**"JUNE[RET]**
**"JULY[RET]**
**"AUGUST[RET]**
**"SEPTEMBER[RET]**
**"OCTOBER[RET]**

Your worksheet should look like Figure 7.5. You should have the titles across the top and the months down the side. GO TO C2, set the auto-advance for the cursor downward by pressing the down arrow key once. That should put your cursor in cell C3. If auto-advance is "off" turn it "on."

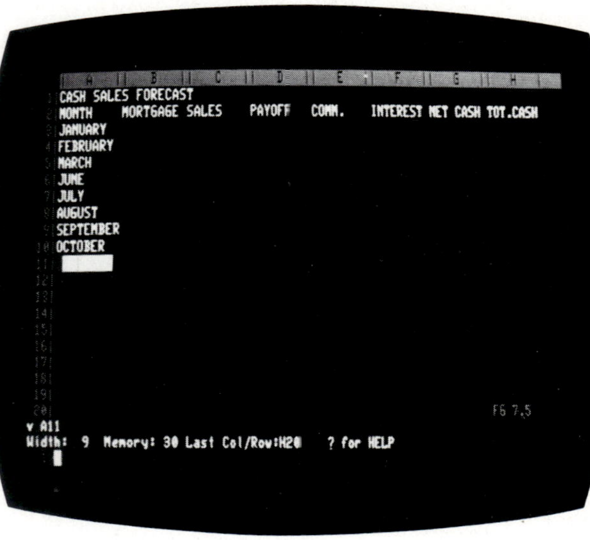


**Figure 7.5** Worksheet headings

You can now begin entering the sales of the various pieces of property. Type

**125000[RET]**
**275000[RET]**
**160000[RET]**
**283000[RET]**
**365000[RET]**
**425000[RET]**
**1673000[RET]**
**518000[RET]**
**227000[RET]**
**351000[RET]**
**=A1[RET]**

It is a little difficult to determine whether the figures you have just entered are under Sales or Payoff, so format everything text right. The instructions are FORMAT, GLOBAL, Text Right. Enter

**/FGTR[RET]**

Now the heading in A1 is strange, so correct it by changing the Format in row 1 to Text Left. Enter

**/FR1[RET]**
**TL[RET]**

Your worksheet should now look like Figure 7.6. You could also spread the data out by enlarging the size of the cells, but that would mean the last column on the screen, H, would then be off the screen

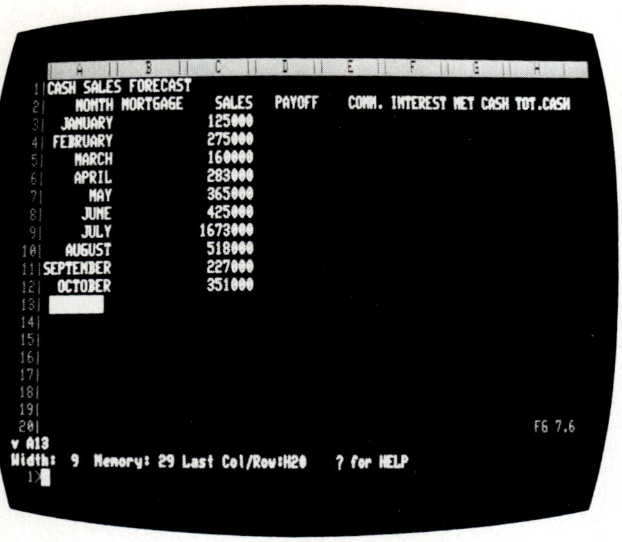


**Figure 7.6** Formatted months and sales

when column A is on the screen. Since you want to be able to see the entire worksheet at once, we'll leave it as is.

Remember, we said that the property is sold on the last day of the month. That's the day you get your money. Therefore the mortgage amount for January is the mortgage on all of the properties listed in column C. To determine the mortgage, multiply the total times 65%. In order to get this amount, GO TO B3 and enter the formula:

**SUM(C2:C12)*.65** RET

This instructs the program to add all the values from C2 through C12 and to multiply that value by .65. Your value in B3 should be 2,861,300. If the B3 figure on your worksheet does not agree, the most likely place for an error is in entering the sales in column C. Check especially to see that you entered 1,673,000 in C9 rather than 167300. To figure out how much mortgage you'll have at the end of February, subtract the January payoff (65% of January sales) from the January sales. For convenience, you will deal only with dollars. With figures this large, the cents only clutter up the worksheet.

To do this, you will use another new function, INT, which stands for integer (an integer is a whole number, i.e., the integer of 6.2 is 6 and the integer value of 6.74 is 6, the integer of −7.4 is −7 and the integer of −7.9 is −7). This function returns the integer value of an expression. For example, in D3, to arrive at the payoff for January, you will enter a formula that multiplies the January sales value (125,000) by .65 and you will ask for the integer of that value. Be sure your cursor is in D3 and enter

**INT(C3*.65)** RET

Your value in D4 should now be 81250. You will need this same formula (adjusted to each cell) for all of column D, so use the REPLICATE command. Replicate from D3 to D4 through D12. Enter

**/RD3** RET
**D4:D12** RET

You are ready to enter the February mortgage amount. GO TO B4. The February mortgage is the January mortgage (B3) minus the January payoff (D3). Enter

**B3−D3** RET

Because you will need this formula to calculate the mortgage for each month, replicate from B4 to B5 through B12 by entering:

**/RB4** RET
**B5:B12** RET

Your worksheet should now look like Figure 7.7. The next thing to compute is the formula for

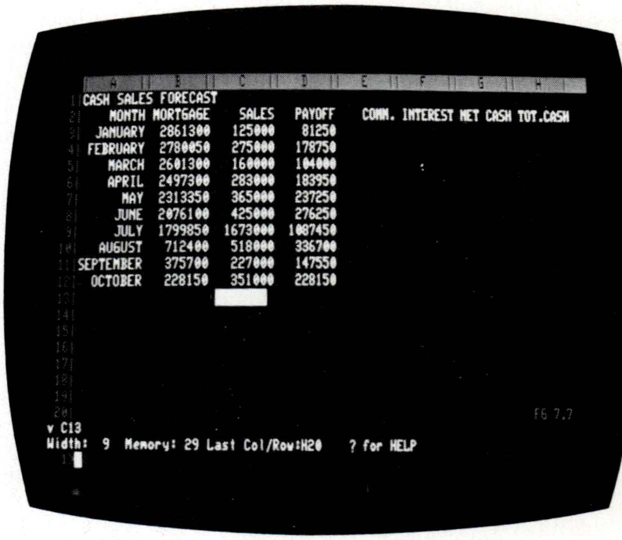


**Figure 7.7** Mortgage calculations

Sales Commissions in E3. Enter the formula in E3, and let's go through it to determine what it does:

**IF(C3<200000,(C3−100000)*.05+6000,(C3−200000)*.04+11000)**

First of all, IF C3 is less than 200000, the program evaluates the first expression after the comma. The first expression after the comma is (C3−100000)*.05+6000. The sales commission you have to pay on the first $100000 is 6% or 6000. The formula begins by subtracting that 100000 from the total sale and then multiplies the difference by 5%. The 6000 is then added to the total. In this instance, the sale value is 125,000 so the program subtracts 100000 from 125000 and multiplies the result (25000) by 5%. This gives you a total of 1250. Add 6000 to 1250 and you have 7250. Enter the formula in E3 and see if the total there is 7250.

This use of the IF conditional is more complex than the example used in Chapter 6. Here, the IF function provides for conditional computations and operates on three comma-separated formulas between the far left and right parentheses. The first formula is the conditional test to be performed (IF C3 is less than 200000). The second formula is calculated if the conditional formula is true, and the third formula is calculated if the first conditional formula is not true.

What would happen if the amount had been more than 200000? That's what happens in E4. The program skips the second expression (C4−100000)*.05+6000, subtracts 200000 from C4(275000), then multiplies the remainder by 4% and adds 11000. Why 11000? Because it is the total of 6% of the first 100000 and 5% of the second 100000.

Rather than typing in that whole formula in each of the column E cells, replicate from E3 to E4 through E12. Enter

**/RE3**RET
**E4:E12**RET

Are the sales commissions what you expected they would be? Your results should be the same as Figure 7.8. The important thing to keep in mind for complex IF statements, or any other function for that matter, is that they are logical. If you were doing this manually, you would probably do it in exactly the same manner that you just did it in SuperCalc.

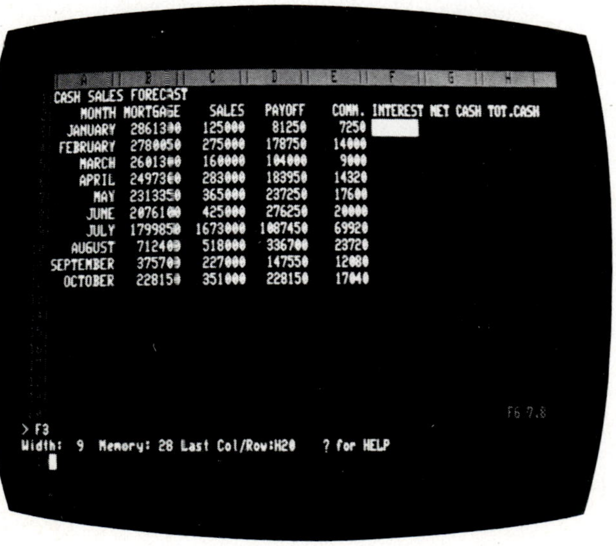


**Figure 7.8** Sales commissions

Now the interest rate. You want to be able to ask an important "what if" question here: What if the prime rate changes? As you know, it fluctuates a lot. Although you can't predict what it will be, you can make some allowances for it. You'll make another entry at the top of the worksheet. GO TO D1 and enter

**"PRIME INTEREST RATE=**

GO TO G1 and type

**16.25**

Then GO TO F3 and multiply the interest rate by the mortgage. To do this, enter

**INT(((G1+2)/1200)*C3)**RET

The value in F3 should be 1901. In the expression, G1+2 is the interest rate plus 2. You can divide this by 12 to get the monthly interest rate, but that isn't what we've done. For convenience, the prime rate is expressed as 16.25%. This number must be divided by 12 to get the monthly interest rate. Rather than divide the interest rate by 100 (to change it to a decimal rate) and then divide by 12 (to get the monthly rate), we chose to multiply first. This is a good way to cut down on the number of multipliers inside your formula. The last thing the program does is multiply the monthly interest by the mortgage amount.

Once again you will want this formula for February through October, so use the REPLICATE command. This time, however, you will make a few changes in this command. Begin by entering the REPLICATE command and indicate that you want to start at F3:

**/RF3**RET

When you enter the "To" range, type F4:F12 but also ask for Options by pressing the comma (,):

**F4:F12,**RET

The computer will respond

**N(o Adjust), A(sk for Adjust), V(alues)**

The A(sk) option lets you specify what type of formula adjustments will be made. You want the calculations based on the interest rate in G1, so the formula needs to be adjusted. Enter

**A**

The program then will ask

**Source cell F3. Adjust G1 (Y or N)?**
**Replicating . . . F**

No, you do not want G1 changed because that is the interest rate. Respond no by typing:

**N**

Then it will ask if you want to adjust C3. Adjusting C3 will make the mortgage amount relative, and you do want those adjusted. To reply yes, type

**Y**

Your display should now look like Figure 7.9.

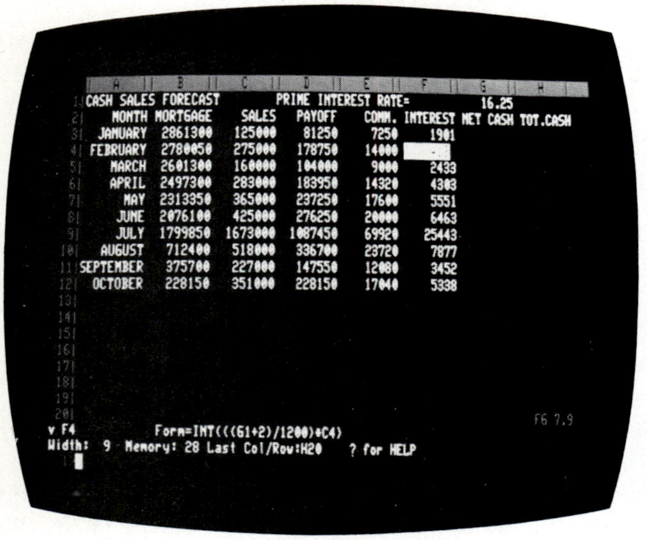


**Figure 7.9** Computed interest rates

The next category is Net Cash. This is Sales (C3) minus Payoff (D3), minus Commission (E3), minus Interest (F3). To enter this in G3, type

**C3−D3−E3−F3**[RET]

Now, replicate from G3 to G4:G12 by entering:

**/RG3**[RET]
**G4:G12**[RET]

Your worksheet should now look like Figure 7.10.

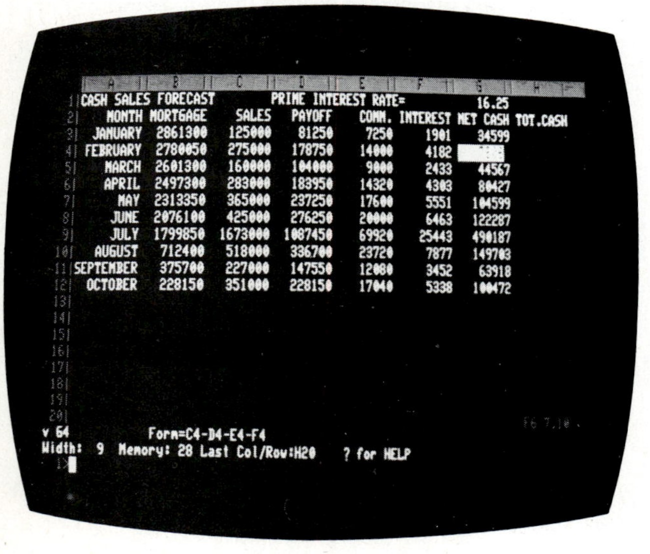


**Figure 7.10** Net cash value

The Total Cash received in the end of the first month (January) is the same as the value in G3. So, in H3 where the total of accumulated cash is calculated, enter

**G3**[RET]

Now, in H4, figure the Total Cash for the rest of the months. Add each month's Net Cash to the previous month's Total Cash. Enter

**H3+G4**[RET]

Replicate this by typing:

**/RH4**[RET]
**H5:H12**

Your worksheet should look like Figure 7.11. It shows that you made a tidy sum in your real estate transactions, even in times of very high interest rates!

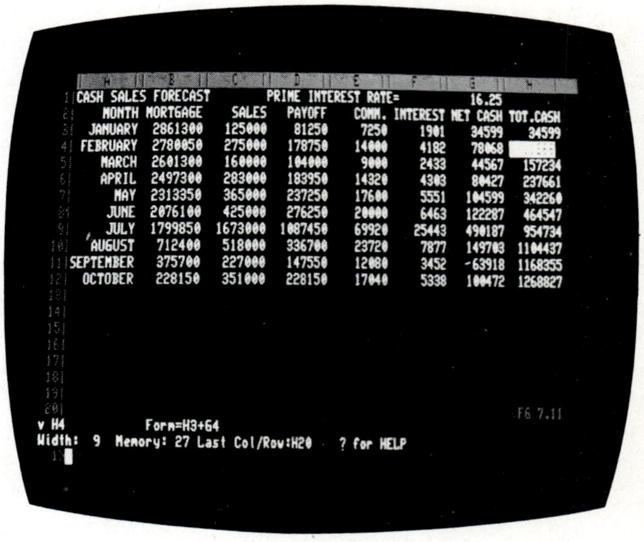


**Figure 7.11** Total cash calculations

## NET PRESENT VALUE

Financial forecasting has value for personal decision making as well as for business decision making. Let's look at a particular example. Assume that your daughter will begin attending college in one year and that you would like to give her something that she can cash in at the beginning of each of her undergraduate years to pay some of the tuition costs. One way to do that is to buy discounted bonds that will mature one a year for four years, beginning in one year. Suppose you want to provide her with bonds that will have a $2000 value and arrange it so that she cashes in one each year. You will need four of the bonds. Assume that the bonds have an interest rate (discount rate) of 8%. How much should you pay for the bonds?

The accounting method used in determining this is called *Net Present Value*. Net Present Value is computed using the following formula:

**B/(1+R)**N**

In this formula, B is the future benefit you expect to derive from the bond purchase, R is the interest or discount rate and N is the number of periods until maturity. The ** means "1+R raised to the Nth power." The Net Present Value (NPV) of $2000 discounted at 8% to be received in one year, then, is 2000/1(1.08). This means that you should pay $1904.76 for a one year 8% bond with a $2000 face value (if you find the 8% rate acceptable in the first place).

The NPV for the $2000 bond that will mature in two years is 2000/(1.08)(1.08) or 2000/(1.08)**2 which is $1714.68. In order to find out how much you need to invest today in order to provide your daughter with $2000 in bond redemptions, you could set up a worksheet and figure each bond's price, then total the value and arrive at a price for the four bonds. There is, however, another way in SuperCalc. It has a built-in function called NPV or Net Present Value. The general format for NPV is as follows:

**NPV (discount, range)**

In our example, the discount will be 8%. The range will be the cells where the bond values are stored. ZAP your worksheet (save anything you want to keep first, however) and put the cursor in A1. Then type

**2000**

Replicate this figure into A2 through A4 by typing

**/RA1** RET
**A2:A4** RET

That should put the bond value of $2000 in A1 through A4. Then move to B1. In B1, you will enter the NPV formula that will tell you how much you should spend for the bonds. Enter

**NPV(.08,A1:A4)** RET

The figure in B1, $6624.25, indicates the amount you should pay for the bonds. NPV assumes you have something of value that will be redeemable later, that there is one discount rate or interest rate for all, and that the period between redemptions will be the same for all of them. That is, if the first one will be redeemed in one year, the next will be redeemed one year later, and so on. The NPV function may not fit your particular calculation needs, but when you have one discount rate to deal with and equal redemption periods, it can save a lot of time and effort.

This ends the Tutorial Section of the book. If you have arrived at this page after working through all the exercises and examples in the Tutorial Section, congratulations! You should be able to use SuperCalc effectively in your own areas of application now. The Tutorial Section has dealt with all the commands available in SuperCalc and most of the built-in functions. There are so many options to the commands, however, that you will probably want to look through the Reference Section carefully to look at some of the less commonly used options. The ones we use less often may be the very ones you find most useful. In addition, there are several built-in functions which have not been mentioned. ABS, for example, returns the absolute value of a number. If A1 contains −34, and ABS(A1) is in C3, then C3 will contain the value 34. There is also a function that computes the mean of a group of cells (AVERAGE), several functions based on Boolean algebra (AND, OR, NOT, and IF), trigonometric functions, log functions, and others. See Chapter 10 in the Reference Section for more detail on all the functions.

# REFERENCE SECTION

## Chapter 8

# Entering Data: Numbers, Text, and Formulas

The Reference Section of this book has two purposes: (1) to provide a quick overview of how to use the SuperCalc commands and functions, and (2) to give detailed information on each operation. If you need to review which command to use, or the use of a particular function, this is the place to look. Also, the screen displays illustrated in this section will help you see how your screen should look after entering various commands and performing different functions.

To help you look up information a little easier, this section is divided into 3 chapters. In this chapter, we will show you how to enter data. Chapter 9 explains all the commands used in SuperCalc. Chapter 10 discusses the built-in functions.

### WHERE TO FIND IT . . .

Below is a list of the main topics covered in Chapter 8 and the page number on which they are discussed:



### HOW TO USE THE REFERENCE GUIDE

If you have read the Introduction and Tutorial Sections, you have seen examples of how SuperCalc is used in a variety of settings. Perhaps you have worked through the examples in the Tutorial Section. In fact, examples have been used extensively in the book and will occasionally be used in the next three chapters. More often, however, screen displays will be used to show how your screen should appear for a particular operation.

**Things to Look For**

Also in this section you will see red boxes. Inside these boxes will be terms, commands or functions. The boxes will act as cues to let you know what is coming. An explanation of the material in the box follows each red box; just as there was a box followed by this brief description.

## LOADING SUPERCALC

Before we present material on entering data, it is important to know how to get SuperCalc running on your machine. The appendix contains a detailed description on making backup copies and how to format diskettes. If you have questions on how to get SuperCalc into your system, please review the appendix. Briefly, once CP/M is loaded in the computer, the screen will read

**NAME OF YOUR COMPUTER SYSTEM**
**XXK CP/M 2.21**

A>

The screen will display the name of your particular system, the fact that XXK of memory is available in the system, and the version of CP/M that you have (ours was 2.21, yours may be 2.27 or something else). Once you have this on the screen, you are ready to load the SuperCalc program. After the A> enter

**SC** RET

The SC stands for SuperCalc. When you press the key marked **RETURN** (**ENTER** on some systems), the computer reads the SuperCalc program from the diskette and puts it in the computer's memory. The screen changes to read:

**SuperCalc(tm)**
**Version 2.21**
**Terminal: Your System**
**CPU: Your System**
**S/N- CP/M 2.21**
**Copyright 1982**
**SORCIM CORP.**
**Santa Clara, Ca.**
**Enter "?" for HELP or "return" to start.**

Again, your version number may be different, and the terminal as well as the CPU will be tailored to your system. The serial number is exclusive, and the CP/M version may or may not be the same. The important part right now is the last line. If you are ready to start SuperCalc, press RET and a blank worksheet like the one in Figure 8.1 will be displayed.

## SUPERCALC SCREEN DISPLAY

### Entry Line

When SuperCalc is loaded into your system, there are 3 lines at the bottom of the screen:

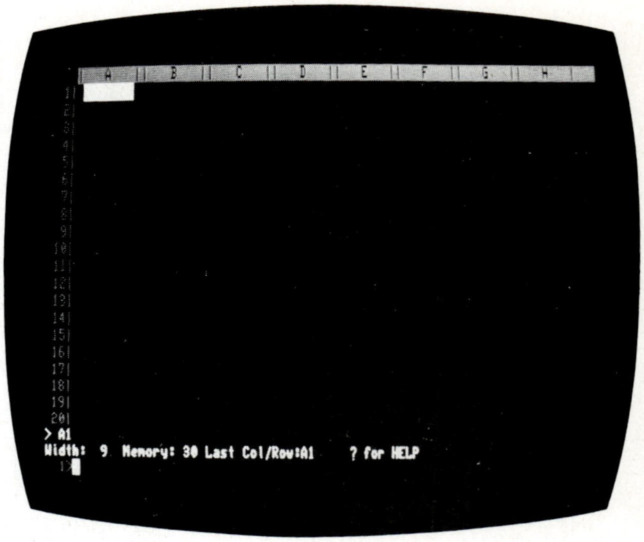


**Figure 8.1** A blank SuperCalc worksheet

**>A1**
**Width: 9 Memory: 30 Last Col/Row A1**
**? for HELP**
**1>**

The last line—the one with the number one and a greater than symbol (>)—is the entry line. The entry line is where you put information on the worksheet. Through data typed on the entry line, you tell SuperCalc how to label columns and rows (text), what numbers to put in each cell (data), and how to put those numbers together to perform computations (formulas). There is more information on the entry line in Chapter 9.

### Prompt Line

The next to the last line is called the prompt line. Normally, it displays four things: (1) the present width of the active cell (actually the width of the current column in which the cursor is located); (2) how much memory, or room for additional material, is left; (3) the last column and row where you worked; and (4) the Help Key. An example of this line is

**Width: 9 Memory: 33 Last Col/Row: J10 ? for Help**

**Width: 9**

This is the column width of the active cell, and the default setting is 9. This can be changed globally, that is, throughout the entire worksheet, or for specific columns. See Chapter 10 for details on how to change the column width.

**Memory:33**

This shows how much memory is available to you in *kilobytes* (a kilobyte is 1024 bytes). This number becomes smaller as you add data to your worksheet or longer if you delete data from your worksheet.

**Last Col/Row: J10**

This gives you the last cell in which you entered either words, numbers, or formulas.

**? for Help**

The question mark (?) reminds you of the availability of the Answer Key. You can press the Answer Key (?) at any time and the SuperCalc program will give you an explanation of your choices at that point. Figure 8.2 displays the screen when the ? is pressed.

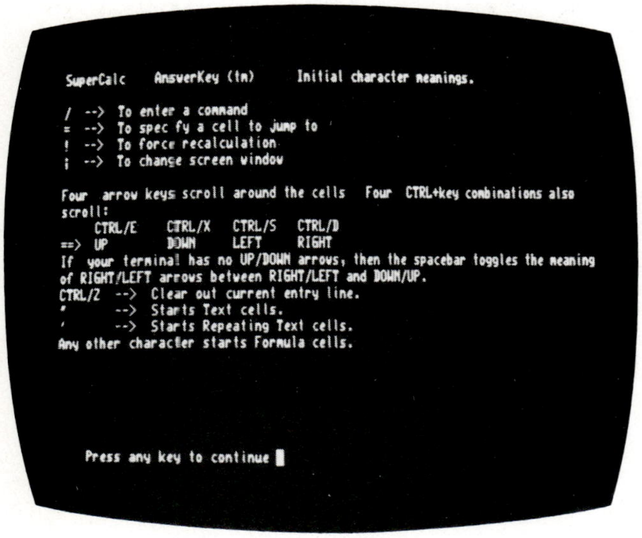


**Figure 8.2** The Answer Key

## Status Line

The status line is the third line from the bottom. It begins with one of the symbols: >, ∧, <, or ∨. The symbol lets you know the direction of the cursor on the worksheet. The cursor automatically moves to an adjacent cell when the RET key is pressed. The direction it will move is indicated by the symbol on the status line. For example, in the status line below, the cursor direction is to the right and the active cell is A1.

**>A1**

If you want to move down, you can change the direction by pressing the down arrow key. To move to the left, press the left arrow key, and to move upward, press the up arrow key.

The status line also tells you other things about the active cell (the cell in which you're currently working). This other information includes: active cell location, that cell's specific format (and whether it is protected), the textual contents of the active cell, and error messages.

Here is an example of a status line:

**<A5 L$TR P Text=February FORMULA Error**

Here is what it means:

**<** The current direction of the worksheet cursor is to the left. Direction is set by the last arrow key pressed. It may be >, <, ∧, or ∨.

**A5** The active cell location. Any information entered is placed in the active cell. In this example, the active cell is A5.

**L$TR** These are the format settings specific to the active cell, numbers are left-justified (L) and in dollar ($) format, and text is right-justified (TR). Detailed information for these settings is given in Chapter 9 under Format.

**P** The P shows that the active cell is protected. If a cell is protected, no information can be entered into it and any contents already in the cell cannot be altered. This space in the status line is blank if the cell is not protected. See Chapter 9 for instructions on how to protect as well as how to unprotect, a cell.

**Text=February** This shows the contents and the type of information in the active cell. See Text and Data in this chapter for more information.

**FORMULA Error** This message indicates there is something wrong with the text that was entered. If there had not been an error message, then nothing would appear on the extreme right side of the status line.

## Text, Numeric Data, and Formulas

In the SuperCalc program, there are three types of information you will want to put on your worksheet: numeric data, formulas and text. This portion of the chapter defines these three types of material and provides examples of each.

## Text

Text refers to the words used on your spreadsheet. For example, the phrases "June Sales" or "Monthly Payment" are text. Generally, anything that can't be added together (e.g., not numbers) and isn't a formula (e.g., G5+4) is text. When text is entered in a cell on the worksheet, it must be preceded by a single set of quotation marks ("). For instance, to enter the phrase, Sample Worksheet, in cell A4, it must be typed

**"Sample Worksheet** [RET]

If the "active cell" is A4, the phrase is displayed there. Text is normally displayed with the letters beginning on the left side of the cell (left-justified), but may be changed to place the last letter on the extreme right of the cell (right-justified). In Figure 8.3, the text in column A is at the default left justification setting, but column B (which contains the same text) has been changed to right justification. See Chapter 9, the FORMAT comand, for more detailed information on how to change justification.

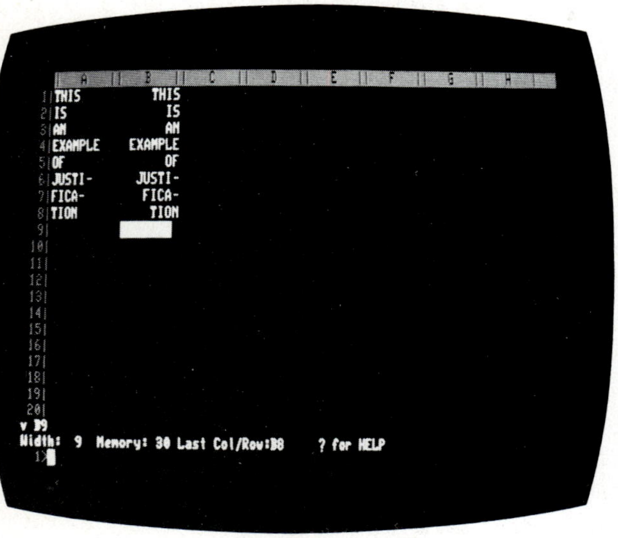


**Figure 8.3** Left and right justification

If the text is too long to fit into a cell, SuperCalc will spill it over into the next cell(s) to the right if it is empty. If the next cell(s) contains any type of information, however, SuperCalc will display as much of the text as possible without disturbing the occupied cells.

## Numeric Data

As used here, numeric data refers to numbers that are either positive or negative (+, −). Numbers are considered positive unless specifically designated as negative.

| Positive | Negative |
|---|---|
| 4 | −7.3 |
| 10.0934 | −6 |

Numbers can have up to sixteen digits plus a decimal point and sign:

−12.34567890123456

Numbers can also be entered in scientific notation. These numbers may have a 16 digit mantissa and a two digit exponent in the range −64 to +63. Thus the maximum range of scientific exponent numbers is

−9.999999999999999 E −64 to
9.999999999999999 E 63

In calculations, SuperCalc automatically switches to scientific notation when a number exceeds its ordinary range or column format. Example: Exp(40)= 2.354e17 in a 9-character wide column.

Although text must be preceded by quotation marks when entered, numbers are not.

## Formulas

Formulas are instructions to add, subtract, multiply and/or divide numeric data. The following symbols are used to designate the various arithmetic operations:

- \+ addition
- − subtraction
- * multiplication
- / division
- ∧ raising to a power

Formulas can use values (numbers) from other cells or built-in functions (built-in functions are operations that SuperCalc will automatically perform when given the necessary instructions; see Chapter 10 for detailed information). Formulas can have up to 116 characters and the result can be seen on the screen as either right- or left-justified. The standard format, however, is for left justification, just like text. The results of formulas, numeric data, are displayed right-justified. See Chapter 9 for instructions on how to set up formulas for right justification.

The following are examples of formulas:

4+3+7
A4+3*7
A4+G3/7−B2
A4+(G3+K7)/7−(B2*8)

There are two terms that are helpful in using formulas: expressions and range. Formulas are sometimes called expressions and often involve specific ranges of cells. Below is a more detailed discussion of expression and range:

## Expressions

Expressions are numeric problems to be solved. It may be a very simple math problem such as 6+2, or it may be an algebraic problem such as 2B/X1−.013K. The expression may have parentheses such as 5*(A1+6)−R2 or even several parentheses such as ((B3+F4)+(09/8+.2))*−8. The math operations required to evaluate the expressions are carried out in a specific order. Expressions are carried out from left to right with ∧ being performed first, * and / performed next, and + and − performed last. In the expression, 4*6/4+2−8, the answer is 0 because 4*6=24, 24/4=6, 6+2=8, and 8−8=0. If parentheses are included, operations within parentheses are evaluated first, then the rest of the equation from left to right. So, if the expresson reads 4*6/(4+2)−8, then 4+2=6, 4*6=24, 24/6=4, and 4−8=−4. Clearly, the results are quite different when the parentheses are added! Expressions can also include functions, which are discussed in Chapter 10.

## Range

A range is part of a row, D6:J6, or part of a column, F2:F8. The range of D6:J6 includes cells D6, E6, F6, G6, H6, I6, and J6. The range F2:F8 includes cells F2, F3, F4, F5, F6, F7, and F8. See Chapter 5 for a detailed explanation of range. Note that C4 is also a range, even though it specifies only one cell.

## Editing the Entry Line

What happens if you are typing information on the entry line and you make a mistake? There are several ways to correct the error. If the material has been entered into a cell, the EDIT command is the feature to use (see Chapter 9). If, however, the information is still on the entry line (you haven't pressed [RET] yet) you can use the back arrow key to move the cursor over to the mistake and retype the material. This can get to be rather time consuming and tedious, however. Another option is to use the arrow keys for editing. For example, suppose you enter the words:

**WOUNDERFUL ENCOUNTER**

and before pressing [RET] realize that the quotation marks are left out and that the word "wonderful" is spelled wrong. Rather than retyping the entry, use the back arrow key to back the cursor over to the letter W. Now, you want to insert the quotation marks, so press the up arrow key. Pressing the up arrow key will move the material on the entry line to the right and insert a space to the left of the cursor. When the space appears, enter the quotation marks. Next, to correct the spelling error, you want to take out the U in WOUNDERFUL. Position the cursor over the U and press the down arrow key. The U disappears. The up arrow makes room to insert a character to the left of the cursor, and the down arrow deletes the character under the cursor. This feature is especially helpful when you enter a long formula and discover an omitted parenthesis or number.

## Error Messages

The last part of this chapter deals with errors that are likely to occur when entering text, numerical data, and/or formulas. All error messages appear on the right side of the status line and are somewhat self-explanatory. Here we will discuss only the error that is likely to be seen in the early stages of using SuperCalc (e.g., errors that are a result of improperly entering text, numerical data, and formulas). Errors that might appear when using commands can be found in Chapter 9. There is actually only one Error Message you are likely to encounter when entering text, numbers, or formulas into a cell:

**FORMULA ERROR**

This message will appear if you have entered text on the entry line without a set of quotation marks ("). For example, suppose you enter

**This is my worksheet[RET]**

(The [RET] means "press the **RETURN** or **ENTER** key.") On the extreme right side of the status line

**FORMULA ERROR**

will appear. Any time material entered doesn't begin with quotation marks, SuperCalc expects numbers or a formula. Obviously, there are no numbers in the phrase above, and it is not a formula, so SuperCalc lets you know there is an error. To correct this, use the back arrow key to move the cursor back over your entry, and type

**"This is my worksheet[RET]**

Your text will be entered in the active cell.

The Formula Error will appear any time text has been entered incorrectly. This message will also be displayed whenever there is something wrong with the way a formula has been entered. If you enter a formula and this message appears, check the entry line to make sure you have the correct number of parentheses, commas and/or computational symbols entered properly with no imbedded spaces. For example, if you enter

**A4+G7(H9+C3[RET]**

you will get an error because the rightmost parenthesis is missing (every left parenthesis must have a corresponding right parenthesis and vice versa). Or, if you enter

**A4+G7(H9;C3)** RET

you will get an error because H9;C3 has no meaning. On our system, the plus sign (+) is entered by using the shift key and the semicolon key. In this example, the shift key was not pressed and the semicolon was displayed instead of the plus sign. The entry should be A4+G7(H9+C3). Error messages reflect human mistakes and they are usually easily fixed. Other error messages will be discussed at the end of Chapter 9.

# Chapter 9

# SuperCalc Commands

A *command* is an instruction SuperCalc understands and acts upon. You tell SuperCalc that a command is coming by typing a / at the beginning of the entry line. SuperCalc then lists the one letter abbreviations of all the commands it understands on the prompt line, and you indicate which one you wish to use by typing the one letter code. As the one letter code is typed, SuperCalc spells out the full name of the command on the entry line (e.g., you type /B and SuperCalc displays /Blank). Then SuperCalc prompts you for any additional information that will be needed to execute the command you have selected.

This chapter of the Reference Section describes the instructions or commands that make SuperCalc work for you. The commands are presented in the order their abbreviations appear on the prompt line when you type a /. The options for each command are generally presented in the order they appear on the prompt line after you type the one letter abbreviation of the command you want to use. That should make it a little easier for you to find the detailed explanation of a particular command while working with SuperCalc. Below is a list of the commands available in SuperCalc. The page number beside each command indicates the page where the explanation of that command begins.



A description of common errors you are likely to encounter are explained at the end of this chapter. Also included at the end of the chapter is a description of the Help facility. If you type a ? while giving SuperCalc instructions, a screen of helpful information relevant to the command or option you are working with will be displayed.

SuperCalc is very forgiving at the command level. If you enter a command letter, or an option, and change your mind, it is possible to get out of the current entry by using the left, or back arrow key. In fact, you can "back out" of a command entirely without executing it simply by entering **CONTROL Z** or by pressing the back arrow key until the information on the entry line disappears. Suppose, for example, that you decide to replicate a certain section of your worksheet (e.g., A1 through A6) in another section (e.g., C8 through H8). You would type /R and SuperCalc would ask you for the "From?" range which is A1:A6. Then it would ask you for the "To?" range which is C8:H8. At any point in this process (before you press [RET] after entering C8:H8), you can forget the whole thing by pressing the left arrow key several times. Each time you press the left arrow key, SuperCalc goes back and "undoes" a step in the command execution process. If you press the back arrow several times, SuperCalc will take you back to the point just before you entered the /R command. It's nice to know you can get yourself out of something so easily! As mentioned before, you can also cancel any command by pressing **CONTROL** ([CTL]) **Z.** Hold down the [CTL] key and the Z key at the same time.

Commands, like any other material on the entry line, can be changed using the "in line editor" features of SuperCalc. These features use the arrow keys to edit and correct material on the entry line. Use the left and right arrow keys to move the cursor around on the entry line. If you place the cursor over a character and type another one, the new character replaces the old one. The simplest way (although not usually the fastest) to correct an error is to use the left arrow key to move the cursor to the very beginning of the entry line and then retype the entry. The up and down arrow keys, however, let you do more sophisticated editing. When you press the up arrow key, SuperCalc inserts a space at the location where the cursor is located on the entry line. If, for example, the cursor is on the L in CAL, pressing the up arrow will result in CA L. Now you can type a second L in the inserted space. Pressing the down arrow key deletes the character under the cursor. If the cursor is located on the second A in CAALL, pressing the down arrow will produce CALL since one of the A's will be deleted. Use the up and down arrows as often as necessary to correct and edit material on the entry line. When you are finished, press the [RET] key to enter the material into a cell or to tell SuperCalc you are ready for it to execute a command. If you have edited something and the cursor is not at the end of your typed material, that is not a problem. Even if the cursor is at the beginning of a heavily edited line, SuperCalc will read and respond to everything that is on the entry line.

A few of the commands use only the active cell (the cell where the worksheet cursor is located). Most allow you to specify which cell or cells the command is to affect. Column addresses may be entered as either capital or lower case letters (C1 or c1); SuperCalc will convert lower case letters to uppercase.

If, when SuperCalc requests a location on the worksheet, you want to designate the active cell as the location where the command should be executed, you can press the comma (,). This is a convenient shorthand that saves time. In addition to the comma (,) you can use the **ESCAPE** ([ESC]) key to indicate the current cell. That is, if SuperCalc requires you to specify a cell and the one you want to use is the active cell, pressing the [ESC] key is the same as typing in the cell location. In addition, if SuperCalc asks for a range (see below for explanation of range) of cells, you can press [ESC] to indicate the beginning of the range, then use the arrow keys to move the cursor to the cell that is the end of the range to be specified. If you press the : key when the worksheet cursor is in the cell that specifies the end of a range, SuperCalc will enter the name of that cell on the entry line. You can also terminate the **ESCAPE** format by pressing [ESC] and then the [RET] key. This process, by the way, does not permanently modify the active or current cell. When you finish the current cell is the same as it was before pressing the [ESC] key.

The **RETURN** key ([RET]) is the last key you press to execute a command. It tells SuperCalc you have completed entering a command and its options and are ready for it to follow those instructions. Many commands, however, will execute without the [RET] key being pressed. It depends on whether SuperCalc can tell whether you have entered everything on the entry line that is necessary to execute the command.

## AN EXPLANATION OF RANGE

Most of the commands available in SuperCalc will ask you to specify which cell or cells should be used by the command. Often the term *range* will be used to prompt you for an indication of the cell(s) to be used. The term range covers a multitude of sins. Range is a general term for anything that tells SuperCalc what part of the worksheet is to be acted upon. Here are some more specific terms that identify different types of ranges.

*Cell.* A cell is the basic element of the worksheet. Each cell is an intersection of a row and a column.

Cells are designated by their column (one or two letters) and row (a number) coordinates. A1, B34, R231 and E45 are all cells.

*Row.* A row is a set of cells designated by a number from 1 to 254. Rows of cells run from the left side of the worksheet to the right side. You can see a part of rows 1 through 22 on the screen when SuperCalc begins working (you may have a different capacity screen that shows more or less than 22 rows at a time). Row 1 begins at cell A1 and extends all the way across the worksheet to cell BK1. A command that affects row 1 will act on all the cells in that row, not just the ones you can see on the screen.

*Column.* A column is a set of cells designated by a letter or letter pair from A to BK. Columns of cells run from the top of the worksheet to the bottom. You can see part of columns A through H on the screen when SuperCalc begins working (you may have a different capacity screen that shows more or less than 8 columns at a time). Column A begins at cell A1 and extends down the worksheet to cell A254. A command that affects column A will act on all the cells in that column, not just the ones you can see on the screen.

*Partial Row.* This refers to a portion of a row. You specify a partial row by indicating the beginning and ending points. The beginning and ending cells are separated by a colon. A1:E1 is a partial row that includes cells A1, B1, C1, D1, and E1.

*Partial Column.* This refers to a portion of a column. You specify a partial column by indicating the beginning and ending points. The beginning and ending cells are separated by a colon. A1:A5 is a partial column that includes cells A1, A2, A3, A4, and A5.

*Block.* The term block sometimes refers to a partial row or column. A more complex use of the term, however, defines a section of the worksheet that encompasses a group of cells in several rows and columns. Look at the diagram below:

| | | | |
|---|---|---|---|
| A1 | B1 | C1 | D1 |
| A2 | B2 | C2 | D2 |
| A3 | B3 | C3 | D3 |
| A4 | B4 | C4 | D4 |

The block A1:D4 specifies all sixteen cells in the diagram above. A1, the beginning cell, defines the top and leftmost border of the block, and D4 defines the bottom and rightmost border of the block.

*List.* A list is a mixed bag of cell designations. Some commands let you specify a range like this: (A1,D1:D4,C3). This is a list that includes cells A1, D1, D2, D3, D4, and C3. A list is enclosed in parentheses and can include single cells, partial rows or columns, and blocks.

## SUPERCALC COMMANDS

### B(lank)

This command will Blank, or erase the contents of all unprotected cells in the range given. To Blank a single cell (C7), enter

**/BC7**[RET]

The / tells SuperCalc that a command is coming. Typing the B instructs the program that you want to Blank. After you entered the B, the prompt line changed to read:

**Enter Range**

At that point you could have specified a single cell or a range of cells. For this example, you entered C7. After pressing [RET], the prompt line responded

**Blanking**...

When the command was completed, the screen returned to its previous display with C7 empty. You could have requested that a partial column be blanked by entering that specific range. For instance, to Blank C7 through C12 you would have entered C7:C12 in response to the prompt, Enter Range. That would have blanked cells C7, C8, C9, C10, C11, and C12. You could also have blanked a row. Using Blank to erase C7 through H7 would remove the contents of C7, D7, E7, F7, G7, and H7. To Blank a block of cells (C7 through H12), enter C7:H12 and every cell from column C and row 7 through column H and row 12 is erased. You can blank an entire row by entering its number or an entire column by entering its letter name.

If you have given instructions to format the cell in a particular way, the Blank command will erase those instructions as well as the contents of the cell. See Format in this chapter for more information. Cells protected by the Protect command will not be affected by Blank (see Protect).

### C(opy)

The Copy command is used for making a one-to-one copy of a cell, a partial row, a partial column or a block of cells to a new location of the same size and format. You can use Copy to put the contents of cell A1 in another cell (e.g., E6). If you Copy the contents of A1 to E6, the material will appear in two places, A1 and E6. It is not removed from A1 when the copy is made, it is simply copied.

Copy will also take the contents of a range of cells (e.g., A1:A4) and duplicate or copy those contents in another range of cells. The destination range will be the same size as the originating range. You specify the beginning cell in the destination range and SuperCalc figures out the rest. Copy will copy a partial column to another partial column, a partial row to another partial row, and a block to another block. But it will not copy a partial row to a partial column or a partial column to a partial row.

To use Copy, enter a / and the letter C. After entering /C, the prompt line will request

**From? (Enter Range)**

The program now wants you to tell it which cell or cells you want copied. You can enter a cell (A19), a partial row (A10:C10), a partial column (B6:B9), or a block of cells (A1:C1). For this example, enter

**A1:C1**[RET]

This tells SuperCalc to Copy the data in cells A1, B1, and C1. Next, the computer responds

**To? (Enter Range), then Return; or "," for options**

Remember that Copy makes a one-to-one duplicate of the source into a destination range of the same shape and size. You do not have to indicate the entire range where the copies go, however. All you need to do is specify the cell in the top-left location of the range. SuperCalc will do the rest. Let's say you want to Copy into cells C6, D6, and E6. Enter

**C6**[RET]

Any data in A1:C1 is copied into C6, D6, and E6. A1 is copied to C6, B1 is copied to D6, and C1 is copied to E6.

*The Options for Adjustment*

As long as you are copying text or values (numbers) the Copy command is relatively straightforward. If, on the other hand, you are copying formulas, the plot thickens considerably. Consider the diagram below which describes the contents of a section of the worksheet:

| | A | B | C | D | E | F |
|---|---|---|---|---|---|---|
| 1 | 03 | 05 | A1+B1 | 09 | A1+B1+C2 | |
| 2 | 01 | A1+E1 | 02 | B1+E1 | | |

If you copy A1 to F1 the only effect will be to put the number 3 in cell F1. What will happen if you tell SuperCalc you want to copy C1 to F1? C1 contains the formula A1+B1. If you tell SuperCalc to Copy C1 to F1 and press the [RET] key, it will automatically *adjust* the formula when it is copied. That is, F1 will contain the formula D1+E1. The C1 cell formula added the values in the two cells to the left of it. Unless told to do otherwise SuperCalc will adjust the fomula to be copied so that the formula in F1 adds the values in the two cells to the left of the destination cell, F1. Suppose you don't want the "automatic adjust" feature? You can repress the automatic adjust when the screen displays this prompt:

**To? (Enter Cell), then Return; or "," for Options**

Instead of entering F1 as the destination cell and pressing [RET], type F1 and then a comma:

**F1,**

The prompt line will change to this:

**N(o Adjust), A(sk for Adjust), V(alues)**

If you want the formula copied without adjustment, press N for No Adjustment. In our example, that would mean F1 would contain the formula A1+B1. If you want the value to be copied, but not the formula just type V. The formula A1+B1 produces a value of 8 since 3 is in A1 and 5 is in B1. If the Values option is selected, SuperCalc doesn't transfer the old formula or create a new one. It computes the value of the old formula and puts that number in the destination.

The final option, Ask for Adjustment, is selected by typing A. This option takes each element of the formula and asks you if you want it adjusted. In the example it will ask if A1 should be adjusted. If you type Y it will change A1 to D1. If you type N, the formula in F1 will begin with A1. Then it asks about B1. You can keep it as B1 or have it adjusted to E1. This option is very flexible, but if you have a large section of the worksheet to be copied, with many formulas, it will take quite a while to tell SuperCalc which ones should be adjusted and which should not be adjusted.

The commands Replicate and Load also make adjustments when they are used. You have the same options in them that you do with Copy. The Load command is affected if you load part of a worksheet into a section of the worksheet that is different from its original position. The Delete, Insert, and Move commands automatically adjust formulas affected by their action. There is no option other than "auto-adjust" for these commands.

## D(elete)

The Delete command deletes a row, column or file (a file is data stored on diskette). The Delete command totally removes the row or column specified and moves over everything to the right of the column (or below the row) to replace what was deleted (the command will not execute if the specified row or column contains a protected cell, see Protect in this chapter). After you enter /D the prompt says

**R(ow), C(olumn), or F(ile)**

If you reply R, the prompt becomes

**Enter row number**

You may now enter a number from 1 to 254 or specify the row where the active cell is located by typing a comma or pressing RET. Rows below the deleted row move up and all row numbering is adjusted. If row 4 is deleted, row 5 moves up and becomes row 4 and so on.

If you enter C, the prompt becomes

**Enter column letter**

You may now enter a letter or letter pair or specify the current column where the active cell is located by typing a comma or pressing RET. Columns to the right of the deleted column move left and all column lettering is adjusted. If column D is deleted, column E moves left and becomes column D and so on.

If you enter F, the prompt becomes

**Enter filename (or Return for directory)**

Here you can enter a file name or press RET to see a list (directory) of the files on the diskettes in your disk drives. If you press RET, your worksheet disappears and you see a menu which gives you three choices:

**C(hoose) alternate disk drive**
**D(isk) directory, all files**
**S(uperCalc) format files only**

At the top it gives you the name of the last file that you loaded, your current disk and your current work file.

If you select C, you can change the current work disk (the disk SuperCalc expects to use). If you choose D, the SuperCalc program shows you the files in the directory of your current work disk. To get back to the menu press any key. If you choose S, the SuperCalc program will show you only those names with the ".CAL" extension added to the end of the file name. .CAL is added automatically to the files created by the Save command.

To get back to the worksheet at any time, press CTL-Z and you will return to the Delete command where you stopped.

*Examples of Delete*

To Delete row 12:

**/DR12** RET

To Delete column H:

**/DCH** RET

To Delete a file name "MYFILE":

**/DFMYFILE** RET

To Delete a file name "MYFILE" that is on a diskette in Drive B:

**/DFB:MYFILE** RET

## E(dit)

The Edit command is used to correct or modify the contents of cells. It is somewhat different from the entry line editing features described in the first part of this chapter. The Edit command is invoked by typing:

**/E** RET

The computer will reply with

**From? Enter Cell**
**26>/Edit (into current cell)**

SuperCalc wants you to specify the cell which contains the material to be modified or corrected. Suppose you want to edit cell C6. Put the cursor in cell C6 and type

**C6** RET

SuperCalc will retrieve the material in C6 and display it on the entry line. You can now correct it using the arrow keys to move the cursor and to delete and insert characters. When you finish editing the material press the RET key. The edited material on the entry line will be sent to the active cell, C6 in our example, since, that is where the worksheet cursor is located.

The Edit command can also be used to bring in material from one cell to the entry line and send it, after editing, to another cell. Put the cursor in the destination cell and type in the name of the source cell when SuperCalc asks for the "From?" cell.

If you type a comma or press RET when SuperCalc asks "From?", it will assume you want to modify the contents of the current active cell. Thus, in the example used above, typing a comma would have had the same effect as typing C6.

## F(ormat)

The Format command is used to control the way text, numbers, and formulas appear on the worksheet. You can specify one or more display formats to effect the display of numbers and text, and you can specify column width. After entering /F, the prompt is

**Enter level: G(lobal), C(olumn), R(ow), or E(ntry)**

Here you can specify the display format for the entire worksheet (G), a column (C), a row (R), or a cell or group of cells (E). If you reply C or R, you are asked to specify the column or row; "," will specify the current column or row. If you reply E, you can specify a single cell or a range of cells; that is, a partial column or partial row (e.g., B6:B22).

The next prompt you receive depends on the level of formatting you specified. Level of formatting means either Global (the entire worksheet is affected), Row, Column, or Entry.

A G(lobal) or C(olumn) Format has this prompt:

**Define Formats: (I,G,E,$,R,L,TR,TL,*,D, Column Width)**

A R(ow) or E(ntry) Format has the same prompt, without Column Width because rows and entries have nothing to do with Column Width. At this point, you can enter as many Format options as you wish. You indicate you have finished entering instructions by pressing RET.

Here are the possible format options:

**I** Displays numbers as integers, rounding up or down to convert them to whole numbers. Whenever rounding is necessary, only the result appears in the display. The number 56.49, for example, becomes 56 while 56.51 becomes 57. Although numbers are rounded for display, the actual value of the number entered is used in all calculations.

**G** Displays data in the general or default format with numbers right-justified, text left-justified and numbers too large to fit the cell width in exponential notation.

**E** Displays numbers in exponential form, as numbers multiplied by a power of 10. The number 56.49 is written as 5.649e1 in exponential notation; 555666 becomes 5.5567e5 and −555666 becomes −5.557e5. Numbers are rounded in this format. This does not affect the value for calculations.

**$** Displays numbers in dollar format and rounds each value to the nearest cent. It also automatically adds ".00" to the end of whole numbers. For example, when entering $34.00, it is not necessary to enter the .00. All that is necessary is the 34. SuperCalc will add the cents portion. No "$" is displayed.

**R** Displays numbers right-justified.

**L** Displays numbers left-justified.

**TR** Displays text right-justified.

**TL** Displays text left-justified.

***** Displays numbers in bar graph form. The size of the bar graph is determined by the column width. Here is an example. Set column width to 15 by entering

**/FG15** RET

Now, enter 6, 7, 3, 4, 2, 8, 11, 14, 1, 6 in A1 through A10. To display these numbers in bar graph form, type

**/FG*** RET

You can also display a single row or column in bar graph form by replacing G with R or C followed by the appropriate row or column number.

**D** Default. Sets the format of the worksheet to the "next level up." Format instructions can be given for anything from a single cell to the entire worksheet. Sometimes format instructions for different levels are in conflict. SuperCalc uses a priority system to resolve conflicts. A cell format instruction has first priority, then row, then column, and finally global instructions. A global instrucion will thus only affect the format of a specific cell if there is no other format instruction that deals with that cell.

Another way of looking at this is that cell formating overrides any format for the column or row where the cell is located. Where rows and columns intersect, row formatting overrides. Any of these override the global setting. If you select a default format option, a cell controlled by a cell format instruction will "default" back to the next available format instruction relevant to that cell (e.g., a row format if there is one). A cell whose format is controlled by a column format instruction would be controlled by the global format directions.

**Column Width** Sets the width of columns globally or individually. The column may be from 0 to 127 characters wide.

When your entries are contradictory, the format entered last is the one that is used. For example, say you want to format numbers for Left Justification and in a General display. But you enter Right Left

Integer General. Left will take effect because Right and Left determine justification and Left was the last specification entered. General is used because it and Integer both specify ways numbers can be displayed and General was the last one entered. Right and Integer are ignored.

When SuperCalc first begins running, these global format settings are in effect: general numeric display (G), numbers are right-justified (R), text is left-justified (L), and the column width is 9.

## Global

The Global command is used for selecting options that affect the entire worksheet. After entering /G, the prompt line reads

**F(orm), N(ext), B(order), T(ab), R(ow), C(ol.), M(an.), A(uto)**

Most of these options are *toggles*. That is, the first time you enter them, the spread sheet changes, or toggles (as in switches), from the default to the optional state. If you enter the option again, the spreadsheet will toggle back to the default. These options are defined below:

**F** The Form option changes the screen to display any formulas that may be in cells rather than the values. Formulas are displayed like text, left-justified. To display formulas, /GF is used (Global and Formula). To display cell values again, use the /GF command again. If cell A4, for example, has the formula A3+A2 in it, the default display will show the value of A3+A2. That is, if A3 is 29.42 and A2 is 46.21, then the spreadsheet will display 75.63 in cell A4. If you specify the Formula option, the spreadsheet will display A3+A2 in cell A4.

**N** The Next option turns off the "auto-advance" of the cursor when RET is pressed. This means that the cursor does not advance in the current direction when RET is pressed. This mode is distinguished by the absence of an arrow symbol on the left side of the status line. Like the Global Formula, use the Next option once to turn off the auto-advance and use it again to turn it back on.

**B** The Border option turns on and off the display of the borders (borders are the letters at the top of the worksheet and the numbers down the side). You may want to use this command before you get a printout of your worksheet. Also, it is essential to turn off the borders when using the eXecute command. eXecute will not work if the borders have not been turned off! Each entry of B toggles the borders on or off.

**R, C** Specifying R or C determines the order in which your worksheet is calculated. If you choose R for Row your worksheet is calculated across rows, which means that the formulas in row 1 are calculated first, then row 2, and so on. If C for Column is chosen, the worksheet is calculated a column at a time; the formulas in column A are calculated first, then column B, and so on.

**M** The Manual option lets you enter data into the worksheet without having the formulas recalculated each time information is entered. This is especially helpful when you have a large worksheet or are doing a significant amount of data entry because you don't waste as much time waiting for SuperCalc to recalculate all the formulas and display the results in the proper cells. The exclamation mark (!) must be pressed to get the program to do the calculation.

**A** The Auto recalculation option returns the automatic calculation. Each time new data is entered, SuperCalc recalculates any affected formulas.

## I(nsert)

The Insert command creates a new row or column in which new data can be entered. A new row is entered between two existing rows, and a column between two existing columns. After entering /I, the first prompt is

**R(ow) or C(olumn)?**

If you enter R, the prompt says

**Enter row number**

You may enter a number from 1 to 254. To indicate the current row, you may enter a comma (,) or press RET. This inserts a new row of empty cells between the existing rows. A new row appears *above* the specified row.

To Insert a new row between rows 4 and 5, enter

**/IR5RET**

If you enter C (column), the prompt will be

**Enter column letter**

You may then enter a column designation from A to BK. Again, a comma (,) or the RET key can be used to indicate the current column. This inserts a new column of empty cells between the existing columns. A new column is inserted to the *left* of the specified column. For example, to insert a column between columns D and E, enter

**/ICE**[RET]

and the rest of the worksheet adjusts. Columns move right, rows move down. Text and numbers in rows or columns that have been changed stay the same, but will be in a new row. Formulas, however, are automatically "adjusted" to fit their new location. See the information on automatic formula adjustment under the Copy command for details on formula adjustment. As a simple example of formula adjustment, assume that you have placed the formula C1+C3 in cell C4. If you insert a new column at column C, the material in the old column C will be shifted over to become a new column D. Now the formula, which will be in D4, will say D1+D3. The formula has been "adjusted" to the new location.

### L(oad)

The Load command finds a file with worksheet information in it on a diskette and loads it into the computer so you can work with it. You may load all or part of a worksheet. In addition, you can load part of a worksheet stored on a diskette (e.g., A1:A44) into the worksheet at a location other than the original location (e.g., H1:H44). The Load command is used by typing:

**/L**

SuperCalc will prompt with

**Enter filename (or Return for directory)**

If you know the name of the file you want to load, simply type it in and press [RET]. If the file is not on the system drive (usually drive A) you must specify the drive to be used by typing its letter designation and a colon in front of the name of the file. If the file DEMO is on drive A, you can simply type

**DEMO**[RET]

If DEMO is on drive B, type

**B:DEMO**[RET]

The Load command will only load files that have the .CAL extension on them. If our DEMO file was placed on the diskette using the Save command, it will automatically have the .CAL extension. (See Save for more information.)

Once you provide SuperCalc with the name of the file, it will prompt you this way:

**A(ll) or P(art)?**

If you press A for All, the entire worksheet will be loaded and you will be able to work with it as you would any worksheet. If you press P for Part, SuperCalc will prompt

**From? (Enter Range)**

Type in the range you want loaded (e.g., A1:A44) and press [RET]. A new prompt will appear:

**To? (Enter Cell), then Return; or "," for Options**

You should indicate the area of the worksheet where the partial worksheet is to be loaded. In the example you can tell the program to load A1:A44 into A1:A44 by typing A1 and pressing [RET]. The program will now load the material in A1:A44 on the diskette file name DEMO into cells A1:A44 in the worksheet on the screen. When asked for the "To?" or destination range, you type in the top left cell in the range. SuperCalc then fills in the rest. The Part option of the Load command works much like the Copy command. (See Copy for more details. See also the information on Formula Adjustment under Copy since Load Partial adjusts any formulas in the "From?" range so that they fit the "To" location, unless you tell it not to.) The Load Partial command lets you add a comma after specifying the "To" cell if you do not want an automatic adjustment of formulas. You then have three options—N(o adjustment), A(sk for Adjustment), and V(alues). Again, see Copy for complete details on these options.

Here are some examples of loading files:

To load an entire file named QUARTER from drive A, type

**/LQUARTER**[RET]
**A**

Load part of a file (F4:F25) named INCOME, which is stored on drive B. You want to put the material in cells A5:A26 and you want automatic formula adjustment. Type

**/LINCOME**[RET]
**PF4:F25**[RET]
**A5**

Since you can load more than one partial worksheet into the one you are working with, it is possible to create new worksheets from parts of several old ones.

If you type /L and then forget the name of the file you want to load, you can press [RET] and look at a list of the files on your diskettes. (See the File option under Delete for more information on how to get a directory of files since it uses the same procedure.)

### M(ove)

The Move command moves an entire column or row to another location on the worksheet. A column can be moved to another column location; a row can be moved to another row location. To invoke the Move command, type

**/M**

SuperCalc prompts with

**R(ow) or C(olumn)?**

If you wish to move a column, type C; if you want to move a row, type R. For illustrative purposes, assume you want to move column C to column F. You would type C and the prompt line would say

**From? Enter Column Letter**

Type C since you want to move column C and press [RET]. The prompt will ask

**To? Enter column letter**

Since you want to move column C to column F, press the letter F and [RET]. Now the material in column C is located in column F. Columns D, E, and F shifted over to fill in the empty column left when the contents of column C were removed. The empty column left when column F was shifted to the left is now filled by the material from column C. Here is a simplified diagram that may help you see how this works:

*The worksheet before the move*

| | A | B | C | D | E | F |
|---|---|---|---|---|---|---|
| 1 | 01 | 02 | 03 | 04 | 05 | 06 |
| 2 | 21 | 22 | 23 | 24 | 25 | 26 |
| 3 | TEXTA | B1+B2 | B1+C1 | F1/E1 | D1/3 | E1/3 |

*The worksheet after column C is moved to column F*

| | A | B | C | D | E | F |
|---|---|---|---|---|---|---|
| 1 | 01 | 02 | 04 | 05 | 06 | 03 |
| 2 | 21 | 22 | 24 | 25 | 26 | 23 |
| 3 | TEXTA | B1+B2 | E1/D1 | C1/3 | D1/3 | B1+F1 |

The A and B columns are the same before and after since they are not affected by the move. Column C now contains the material that was in column D. The contents of E1 were shifted to cell D1 and the formula reflects that shift. Column D now contains the material that was in E before the formula adjusted, E contains the material that was in F before, and F contains the material moved from C. The new F column (old C column) has the formula B1+F1 in cell F3. B1 is the same as it was in the old location; C1 became F1 because of the move from C to F.

Some commands, such as Copy and Replicate, allow you to suppress the formula adjustment option. Move, Delete, and Insert do not allow an option. Formulas are always adjusted to new locations.

As with several other commands, you can use the comma or the [RET] key to designate the current column or row. Pressing the [ESC] key will also designate the current column or row. If you use the [ESC] key to specify the "From" column or row, you can move the cursor to the "To" column or row, and press [ESC] to specify the "To" designation.

## O(utput)

This command writes part or all of a worksheet to a printer, terminal, or a diskette. You can write any size of range you wish. If you write your worksheet to a disk file, you can use a system text editor or another editor to add further information or reformat your report before printing. You can also include SuperCalc reports in other documents. A file saved on a diskette using the Output command cannot be used by SuperCalc, however. See Save for instructions on how to put a file on diskette that will be used again in SuperCalc.

When you enter /O you'll notice the prompt line becomes

**D(isplay) or C(ontents) report?**

If you choose D, an exact copy of your displayed worksheet is sent to the printer, terminal, or diskette. The C option tells SuperCalc to list the *content* of the cells in the specified range, rather than the cell values. Each cell is either printed, displayed, or written (depending on what you chose) one line at a time. The information includes the specific cell format, the type of data contained in the cell and the cell contents. Contents outputs the formulas, Display outputs the results or "answer" to the formula.

The next prompt says

**Enter Range**

You can enter any range you want printed, displayed or written to the diskette. (If you want the entire worksheet, type All.) Press [RET] when the range is selected. The prompt line will then ask

**Enter Device: P(rinter), S(etup), C(onsole), or D(isk)**

If you enter C, your file is displayed on the terminal screen or "console." This is useful for double checking your spreadsheet before creating a "hard copy" (i.e., printed) version.

To get a hard copy of your worksheet information, choose option P for Printer. This sends the information you have specified to the printer. The default line length is 132, the default page length is 66. That is, the printer is sent lines of material up to 132 characters long and up to 66 lines of material per page. This format is the standard one for computer generated output, but it may not be the format you want. The Setup option, discussed later, allows you to make any changes you need. If your data exceeds the line length, SuperCalc prints as many columns as it can on one page and the excess columns are printed on another page. When your report exceeds the size of the paper you are printing on, the program prompts

**More. . .(Return to continue or Control Z to stop)**

When you press [RET], the program continues to send information to the printer. If you want to interrupt printing at any time, [CTL]Z stops printing and returns you to the worksheet.

If you want to change the standard setting for printing, enter S for Setup. This clears the worksheet from the screen and displays a menu with more options.

At the bottom of the page a new prompt line appears:

**L(ength), W(idth), S(etup), or P(rint)?**

The menu is actually a definition of the options in the prompt line. The following is a more detailed explanation:

- **L** This option is for changing the number of lines per page. If you specify zero (0), your document will be printed as a continuous form without interruptions between pages.
- **W** This changes the number of characters on each line. This can be from 0 to 255 characters per line.
- **S** This option is for sending special codes to the printer to initiate special functions, such as compressed or expanded type, large type or underlining. The use of this option depends on the particular printer used. In essence, selecting the S option lets you type material on the keyboard that is sent directly to the printer. You can send the printer anything you want. Then, when you are finished, press [RET] and SuperCalc will let you select another option (such as Print).
- **P** This sends the material you specify to the printer. Make sure your printer is properly hooked up and turned on.

The third device to which you can send your worksheet data is the diskette. If you choose D for Disk, the SuperCalc program prompts you for a file name. From here the command acts much like the Save command, except that the file created is a "text" file containing the same information that would be Output to a console or a printer, and has a ".PRN" extension (see Save in this chapter). This file cannot be loaded by the SuperCalc program.

The advantage of creating a text file is that you can use this file within other programs, specifically word processing and text editing programs. You can change the information into a more acceptable form, or incorporate your worksheets in other reports or papers. Or you can just save them to print later using the CP/M print utilities.

The following are examples of using the Output command.

To Output in Display format All of the spreadsheet to the printer:

**/ODALL[RET]**
**P**

To remove borders and output a file named WORK1 to a diskette in drive B:

**/GB**
**/ODADB:WORK1[RET]**

Note: Most of the time, when you print a spreadsheet you will probably want to remove the borders (the letters and numbers across the top and down the left side of the spreadsheet). Use the Global command with the Border option before printing (/GB).

## Protect

The Protect command is used to protect a single cell (e.g., K21), a range (e.g., B1:B31), or a block (e.g., B1:G12) so that whatever data is there cannot be changed or erased. Any formatting instructions that apply are also "protected." When using /P, the prompt is

**Enter Range?**

You may then specify the area to be protected. After a cell, range, or block is protected, several commands (e.g., Blank, Copy, Format, Replicate) will bypass that area. That is, the commands will work around the protected areas, if possible, without disturbing the affected cell(s). Delete will not be executed at all if a specified row or column contains a protected cell. The Zap command, however, can be used to override a Protect command. Some terminals display protected areas in a different intensity or brightness so that you can tell at a glance what is protected.

The following are examples of ways to enter information to Protect cells, columns, rows, and blocks:

To Protect cell J7:

**/PJ7[RET]**

To Protect the partial column J3:J8:

**/PJ3:J8[RET]**

To Protect the partial row K14:Z14:

**/PK14:Z14** RET

To Protect a block:

**/PM2:AK7** RET

## Quit

The Quit command allows you to exit from SuperCalc and return to the operating system. If you want to keep the current worksheet, be sure to Save it before using Quit. Using Quit erases the worksheet from memory; it can be very upsetting if a worksheet is lost accidentally. After entering /Q, the prompt is

**EXIT SuperCalc? Y(es) or N(o)**

If you reply Y, you will be returned to the operating system. If you reply N, you will be returned to the SuperCalc worksheet.

## Replicate

The Replicate command is very versatile and has a number of different formats. Each of the different ways it can be used will be dealt with separately.

*One Cell to One Cell.* You can use Replicate to copy the contents of one cell to another cell. Here is an example:

**/RA1** RET
**D6** RET

After selecting the Replicate command with /R, the program prompts for a source range (From?). You type in A1 and press RET. The program then asks for a destination (To?). If you type in D6 and press RET, the contents of cell A1 will be copied in cell D6. This is identical to the operation of the Copy command.

*One Cell to Many Cells.* You can use the command to copy the contents of one cell into many different cells at once. This is handy when you need to enter the same material over and over again. Replicate lets you type it in one cell and then use the command to get the same thing in many other cells. Here is an example:

**/RA3** RET
**C1:C21** RET

Here you tell SuperCalc that you want to replicate the contents of cell A3 to the partial row of cells included in the range C1:C21. If the word "INTEREST" was in cell A1 before this command was executed, the word "INTEREST" would be in cells C1 through C21 afterward. You can copy one cell into a partial row or a partial column. Just specify the correct destination range when the program asks "To?"

*One Partial Column to Several Partial Columns.* If you have something in cells A1 through A5 that you also want in cells E6 through E10, F6 through F10, and G6 through G10, Replicate is the way to do it. Type

**/RA1:A5** RET
**E6:G6** RET

You specify the originating partial column right after typing /R. In this case it was A1:A5. Then you press the RET key. SuperCalc asks for a "To?" range next. You only need to specify the *top* of the range of cells where the replication will occur. In this example, the top range began at E6 and extended across the worksheet to G6. When you press the RET key, SuperCalc finds E6 and replicates the contents of A1:A5 into E6 through E10. Then it moved to F6 and replicated A1:A5 in F6 through F10. Finally, it moved to G6 and did the same thing again. Remember, in the "To?" range you will specify the top leftmost cell in the replication range first and the top right most cell in the replication next, after a colon.

*One Partial Row to Several Partial Rows.* If you have something in cells A1 through F1 that you also want in cells B6 through G6, B7 through G7, and B8 through G8, Replicate is the way to do it. Type

**/RA1:F1** RET
**B6:B8** RET

You specify the originating partial row right after typing /R. In this case it was A1:F1. Then you press the RET key. SuperCalc asks for a "To?" range next. You only need to specify the *left* of the range of cells where the replication will occur. In the example, the top range began at B6 and extended down the worksheet to B8. When you press the RET key, SuperCalc finds B6 and replicates the contents of A1:F1 into B6 through G6. Then it moves to B7 and replicates A1:A5 in B7 through G7. Finally, it moves to B8 and does the same thing again. Remember, in the "To?" range you will specify the top left most cell in the replication range first and the bottom left most cell in the replication range next, after a colon.

Replicate and Copy are similar commands. Both can copy one cell to another cell. Replicate, however, can make "one to many" copies while Copy cannot. Copy, on the other hand, can copy one block of cells to another block while Replicate cannot deal with blocks at all.

### *The Issue of Formula Adjustment*

When Copy and Replicate take data from one cell and move it to another, the cells that contain formulas are adjusted to fit the destination. See the Copy command in this chapter for details on Formula Adjustment. You can suppress the automatic adjustment of formulas by typing a comma after entering the "To?" range. SuperCalc will then give you several options. Again, see Copy for details.

## Save

This command stores the contents of the worksheet on a diskette. Your spreadsheet is written to a diskette under a name you assign. The options give you a choice of saving all of the contents of your worksheet or just the values (e.g., the text and numbers in the cells but not the formulas). After pressing /S, the prompt line reads

**Enter File Name (or RET for directory)**

Now enter the name you have chosen for your file. Just any name, however, will not be acceptable to SuperCalc. There are some guidelines to follow in establishing a file name. For example, the name must start with a letter (not a number), and can have from one to eight characters. There can be no blanks, or any of these other characters in the file name: < > . , ; : = +. Also, if you want the worksheet saved on a diskette in a drive other than the primary drive, you must enter the destination drive letter and a colon in front of the file name. SuperCalc will automatically give the file the extension ".CAL". You do not need to enter it as part of the file name.

The next prompt is

**A(ll) or V(alues)**

Entering A specifies that all of the cell contents are to be saved. The V option converts all the formulas to numeric values and saves the numbers. The formulas are discarded as far as the file on the disk is concerned. They will not be there if the file is loaded back into SuperCalc.

Regardless of which you choose, there are some things that are saved on both options: format settings, global options, title locks, window splits, and active cell location.

If you specify the name of an existing file, the program will display the following prompt:

**File already exists: C(hange name), B(ackup) or O(verwrite)?**

If you choose C (change name), the SuperCalc program will allow you to edit or change the file name you have specified to something else.

If you choose B(backup), the extension of the existing file (".CAL") is changed to ".BAK", and the new file is then saved with a ".CAL" extension. Therefore, your old file remains unchanged and becomes a backup.

If you choose O (overwrite), the SuperCalc program erases the old file and creates a new one of the same name with your current worksheet.

For example:

To Save the entire file (All) that you have named MYFILE:

**/SMYFILEA**

To Save, on drive B, the worksheet called MYFILE, Values only:

**/SB:MYFILEV**

## Title

This command "locks" rows and columns into place on the screen display. As an example, let's say that in column A you have titles such as those in Figure 9.1 (a figure similar to one in Chapter 6 on expense accounts) and you want to check the values of column I. If you scroll over to column I, column A will disappear and you may forget the title of the row you wanted to check. Using the Title command, you can lock in place column A, which contains titles. Then, when you scroll over to column I, the information in column A stays in place.

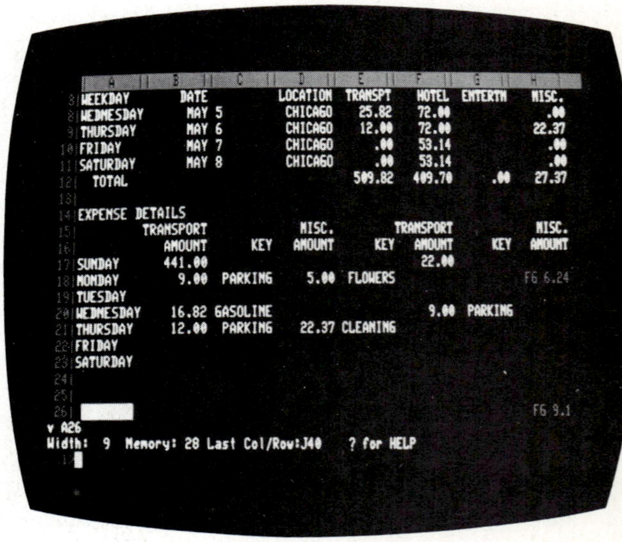


**Figure 9.1** Worksheet with title locks

For example, to use the Title command to lock column A, position the cursor in cell A1 and enter

**/T**

SuperCalc will respond with several options:

**H(oriz.), V(ert.), B(oth), or C(lear)**

The options allow you to specify whether you want to lock titles in a horizontal or vertical direction, both, or to clear the command. The options are

**H** Locks the current row and all rows above it.

**V** Locks the current column and all columns to the left of it.

**B** Locks the current row and column, as well as all rows above and columns to the left.

**C** Clears the title lock.

Because Title uses the current column, your cursor must be in the column you want locked. In this example you want to have all of column A locked, so you place the cursor in A1. You now request a vertical lock by entering:

**V** RET

You can now scroll columns across to column E while A remains in place.

To "unlock" a column or row, you must first use /T and then the Clear option. If you give SuperCalc a new Title command, it replaces any lock you gave earlier.

## Unprotect

Unprotect removes protection from a range of cells and allows the contents or formats to be changed. On terminals that change intensity or brightness in protected areas, notice the Unprotected areas return to regular intensity. Our examples for /Unprotect are the same for /Protect. Review this command to see how the screen looks when something is protected. Examples:

To Unprotect cell J7:

**/UJ7** RET

To Unprotect a partial column (J3:J8):

**/UJ3:J8** RET

To Unprotect a partial row (K14:Z14):

**/UK14:Z14** RET

To Unprotect a block:

**/UM2:AK7** RET

## Window

The Window command will split the screen display into two separate parts. Each portion can have its own format settings and options. Window uses the current row or column. That means the screen will be split at the row or column where the cursor is located. After /W the first prompt is

**H(oriz.), V(ert.), C(lear Split), S(ynch.), or U(nsynch.)**

You have several different ways in which you can divide the screen:

**H** The screen is split horizontally (between rows), with the row that contains the cursor moving down to be replaced by a second border.

**V** The screen is split vertically (between columns), with the current column moving right to be replaced by a second border.

You will notice that when using the Window command, it seems impossible to move from one Window to another. That is, you cannot cross the borders of the Window. You can get from one area to another, however, by pressing the semicolon (;) key. Press it once to move to one window and press it again to return to the other window. While in either section you have all the options available with any commands.

**C** Clears the split screen. The portion that was above or to the left is the "primary" screen; it is now displayed in full.

**S** Synchronizes scrolling in both portions of the screen when the cursor is moving parallel to the split. That is, when you scroll one side of the split screen, the other side of the screen scrolls too.

**U** Unsynchronizes scrolling. The two portions will scroll independently when the cursor is moving parallel to the split.

As mentioned earlier, you can use the Global and Format commands in each of the windows. A Format or Global command you enter in one window does not affect the other one. It is possible, for example, to show the same data with different formats and options; for example, to show the same column as values and as formulas.

## eXecute

SuperCalc allows you (almost) to create a file of commands, store the file on a diskette, and Load/eXecute the file whenever needed. This is a process that is likely to be of interest primarily to advanced users. There are three steps to the process. First, you should decide what commands you want to put in a file and type them into a SuperCalc worksheet *exactly* as you would type them on the entry line. Put each set of directions, up to and including the RET, in a separate cell. For example, put everything in column A, beginning in cell 1 and proceeding down the sheet. When you finish typing in all the instructions, you will have a series of cells with text in them (you must add a " to the beginning of each cell entry to get SuperCalc to accept them). Instructions might be located in cells A1 through A44, for example. You may want to begin your set of instructions with a Zap command (/ZY[RET]) in cell A1. That will clear the worksheet before SuperCalc begins executing the commands in your file.

Now for the second step. Save the file you have created in two ways. If the name of the file is DEMO, save the worksheet, using the Display option, once under the Output command with a .PRN extension. SuperCalc automatically adds .PRN to the name you give your file when the Output command is used. *Remove the borders* of the worksheet before "Outputting" it to disk by typing /GB[RET]. Then, if you give the instruction /ODA1:A44DDEMO, SuperCalc will output the displayed material in cells A1 through A44 to the disk drive using the file name DEMO. It will also change the name to DEMO.PRN. Now you should save the file to disk again using the Save command. Here are the instructions to give for our file named DEMO:

**/SDEMOPAA1:A44[RET]**

This instruction tells SuperCalc to save a program called DEMO using the Part, All options and to save only cells A1 to A44. When Save is used, the extension .CAL is added to the file's name. Thus you will have files DEMO.PRN and DEMO.CAL on your diskette. Should you make a mistake in your list of instructions in the file, you will have to load DEMO.CAL back in and correct the errors. Then you should save the corrected file again. Do it twice, once using Output (see example above) and once using Save.

How do you tell if there are any errors in the file? And how do you use this file you have created? There is a command called eXecute. If you type /X on the entry line, SuperCalc will prompt you for a file name. If you type in DEMO and press [RET], SuperCalc will find DEMO.PRN on the diskette (the one saved using Output). When it finds that file (called a *command file*) it begins with the first set of instructions (in cell A1 in our example) and executes the instructions in the file one by one.

That, at least, is the theory. In fact, most, if not all versions of SuperCalc which were available when this was written would not work at this point. In order to get the DEMO.PRN file to be accepted by the eXecute command you must leave SuperCalc using the Quit command (/QY) and, while in CP/M, rename the file so that it carries a XQT extension. Renaming the file DEMO.PRN so that it becomes DEMO.XQT is done by typing:

**REN DEMO.XQT=DEMO.PRN[RET]**

CP/M will rename the file called DEMO.PRN. It becomes DEMO.XQT, and the eXecute command will accept it now. There are still, however, likely to be problems with getting the file to actually work as expected.

Another alternative is to create a command file like DEMO.PRN in a word processing program or a CP/M editor. Then save the file on diskette, rename it so that it has a QRT extension, and then use the eXecute command. Because SuperCalc reads the file letter by letter, you must be able to send SuperCalc the exact pattern of letters (and codes such as [RET]) that it would receive if you were typing in material from the keyboard. Save this one for a long winter's evening when your spouse is away and the television is broken.

## Zap

The Zap command erases everything from the worksheet, and everything in the computer's memory about the worksheet. In other words, unless the worksheet has been saved, it is gone forever. After entering **/Z**, the prompt from the entry line reads

**/Zap–ENTIRE–Worksheet?**

And the prompt line asks (as if to be sure you want to do this)

**Y(es) to clear everything, else N(o)**

Just remember that nothing remains after Zap is used. Type "Y" if you really want to get rid of everything on the worksheet.

## Answer Key

Just as you can press the ? to get general information on the SuperCalc worksheet, this same key provides more detailed information on aspects of each command. If, after entering the / and a command letter, there is a prompt that is unclear, pressing the ? will produce a display screen to explain various aspects of the command. Suppose that you are about to save your worksheet and have entered /S and the prompt line asks for a file name. What is a file name? Press ? and a screen of information will appear.

A definition for file name is given to help you set one up for saving. At any time in a command, if something is unclear, use the Answer Key (?) to help answer questions.

## ERROR MESSAGES

The error messages discussed in Chapter 8 are probably the ones you'll see most of the time, until, that is, you start using the commands. Fortunately, many of the commands have the same error messages so it is possible that once you've encountered a message, if it comes up again you'll be able to quickly identify the problem. Remember that error messages always appear on the right side of the status line. The error messages discussed here include

- Column ERROR
- Copy ERROR
- Disk Full
- Drive Not Ready
- File NOT on Disk ERROR
- Formula ERROR
- Memory Full
- No Room (at edge) to display window
- Protected Entry
- Range ERROR
- Row ERROR

*Column ERROR.* This message may appear when using Delete, Insert, or Move commands. The program asks if you want to Delete, Insert, or Move a row or column. If you specify a column and enter something besides a letter, this message will appear. Use the arrow keys to correct the error and type in a column letter.

*Copy ERROR.* The message actually reads

**Copy "TO" must be a cell**

When this message is present, it means that more than a single cell has been designated to receive the duplicated material. Copy will put material in more than one cell, but the command expects only one cell when the "To?" prompt appears. See Copy for details.

*Disk Full.* Although diskettes are capable of storing a considerable amount of data, they do have limits. If you get this error, it means you are trying to Save or Output a file that is too big to be put in the space remaining on the diskette. If you have a system with more than one drive, you may be able to put the file on a diskette in another drive. You can also put another diskette in the disk drive and tell SuperCalc to redo the operation. If all else fails, you can tell SuperCalc you do not wish to redo the operation and it will be canceled.

*Drive Not Ready.* You may get this message when you tell SuperCalc to read a file on a drive that does not contain a diskette. To correct the problem, insert the diskette and redo the operation. Disk drives occasionally produce this message and work fine if you tell SuperCalc to try again. If you correct any problems and the drive still isn't ready, you may need to get the computer checked, particularly if you try to use the drive with other diskettes and get the same message.

*File NOT on Disk.* While this can be an alarming message, it usually reflects a spelling error. This is encountered during Load and eXecute commands. First, check to make sure the spelling on the entry line is *exactly* as the file name is on the diskette. Then see if there needs to be a specific disk drive designation. For example, if you saved a file called MYFILE on drive B using the format /SB:MYFILEA[RET], then when you try to load that file, you must enter /LB:MYFILEA[RET]. The computer will not know to look in drive B unless you tell it to do so. If the spelling is o.k., the correct drive has been specified, and the message still shows up, request a directory of file names from SuperCalc to make certain the file does exist. If it isn't on the directory . . . it isn't anywhere.

If this error occurs when you are trying to use the eXecute command, chances are that the ".PRN" extension on the file name needs to be changed. Read the eXecute command discussion in this chapter for information on how that change is made.

*Formula ERROR.* This message appears when text is entered without being preceded by the single quotation mark ("). Just use the back arrow key to go to the beginning of what you typed in on the entry line. Use the up arrow key to create a space, and type in the ". If there are blank spaces anywhere in the formula, uneven numbers of parentheses, or mistakes in typing computational symbols (+, −, *, /), this error will appear. The message is also seen when using the built-in functions if the wrong abbreviation is used (i.e., SQT instead of SQRT) or if blanks are inserted [i.e., SQRT (45) instead of SQRT(45)].

*Memory Full.* A large worksheet may gobble up all the memory available in your computer. You will improve the memory situation if you blank areas of the worksheet you aren't using. Large worksheets can sometimes be broken into two or more smaller ones. That will help.

*No room. . . .* The only time you'll see this message is when using the Window command. This happens when you request a vertical split and the cursor is either in the extreme left column (A) or the extreme right column (BK). If you request a horizontal split and the cursor is at the top of the worksheet (row 1) or at the bottom (row 254), the same message appears. When using Window, remember that SuperCalc uses the active cell as the location for the split. Place the cursor at the location where you want the split to occur. If it is any place on the worksheet besides column A or BK for a vertical split, or row 1 or 254 for a horizontal split, this message will not appear.

*Protected Entry.* If you have a protected range (remember that a range may be one cell, a partial column or row, or a block of cells) and try to use the

Blank, Copy, Delete, Load, or Replicate commands in that area of the worksheet, you will get this message. The Protect command is used to keep any of the above things from overriding material that you don't want changed. If you want to use Blank, Copy, Delete, Load, or Replicate in a protected area, you will first have to use the Unprotect command (see Unprotect in this chapter).

*Range ERROR.* Although there are several types of Range Errors that can appear (i.e., TO must be a partial row; copy won't fit; TO must be a partial column), they all indicate that a wrong range specification has been entered. That is, too many cells or too few or in the wrong column or row. This is probably best remedied by practice with the program and getting used to the terms such as partial column, partial row, cell, block, and range. Generally, if you take a minute to analyze what exactly it is you want to do, and where you want it done, the range will become apparent. To change a range you have already entered, use the arrow keys to edit your entry.

*Row ERROR.* This is just like the column ERROR, except it applies to rows. Found with Delete, Insert, and Move, a row number is needed but something other than a row number has been entered. To correct the problem, use the arrow keys to edit your entry.

This concludes the chapter on SuperCalc commands. If necessary, go over any procedures that are unclear. The next chapter deals with built-in functions.

Chapter 10

# Built-In Functions

To assist you in manipulating data on the worksheet, SuperCalc has several functions which can be performed automatically. For example, if you want to calculate the average or mean of the numbers in cells B6, B7, B8, and B9, you could use the AVERAGE function. AVERAGE(B6:B9) would add up the numbers in cells B6 through B9 and divide the result by 4 (the number of numbers added together). The functions available in SuperCalc make it very easy to perform many complicated calculations easily. Below is a list of the functions and where they are located in this chapter:



Each function is listed on the following pages with a description of how it is used.

**ABS ($)**

Provides the absolute value of the number inside the parentheses. The absolute value of a number is the value without a minus sign:

ABS (−456)=456
ABS (27)=27
ABS (−9.78)=9.78

**AVERAGE (LIST)**

Returns the average of the list or range of cells specified in the parentheses. The "average" calculated by SuperCalc is the mean, not the median or mode. The function adds up the numbers in the cells specified by the list or range and divides by the number of non-blank cells. The result is the Average. If there is a blank cell in the range (e.g., a cell with nothing in it), SuperCalc does not count that cell at all. It will, however, count a cell with a 0 in it. Cells with text are ignored. Here is an example:

A1 contains TEXT B1 contains 2 C1 is blank
D1 contains 4 E1 contains the number 0
F1 contains AVERAGE (A1:E1).

Cell F1 will display the value 2 because SuperCalc added B1, D1, and E1 together, then divided by 3. It ignores A1 because it contains text and C1 because it is blank.

**COUNT (LIST)**

This function returns the number of non-text, non-blank cells included in the list specified in the parentheses. Here is an example:

A1 contains TEXT B1 contains 2 C1 is blank
D1 contains 4 E1 contains the number 0
F1 contains COUNT (A1:E1).

Cell F1 will display the value 3 since there are only three cells (B1, D1, and E1) in the range that are non-text, non-blank cells.

**ERROR, NA**

When SuperCalc encounters any sort of error in a cell it writes "ERROR" in that cell. For example, if you tell SuperCalc to divide A4 by A6 and A6 currently has a 0 in it, that will produce an ERROR in the cell where the A4/A6 is located because you cannot divide by zero. NA stands for "Not Available." It may show up in cells that perform calculations using data from cells that have not yet been calculated. The data is "Not Available." The NA will change when the cell can get all the data it requires to perform the calculations.

You can also place an ERROR or NA message in any cell. Just put the cursor in the cell where the message is to appear, type the message (ERROR or NA) and press [RET].

**EXP (#)**

This function raises "e" exponentially. The number in parentheses is the exponent. Examples:

EXP(2)=$e^2$ or 7.389056
EXP(4)=$e^4$ or 54.59815

**INT (#)**

Returns the integer value of the number in parentheses. The number is not rounded. Examples:

INT(2.5832)=2
INT(45.01)=45
INT(33.99)=33

**LOOKUP (VALUE, COL/ROW RANGE)**

Searches the column or row range specified in the parentheses. It looks for the cell that contains a number which is less than or equal to the value given in the parentheses. When it finds the cell with the number that meets that criterion, it looks in the adjacent row to the right (if searching a column range) or below (if serching a row range) and returns the number located there.

An example would probably help:

A1-45 B1-48 C1-55 D1-75 E1-88 F1-97
A2-43 B2-03 C2-99 D2-67 E2-32 F2-03
Cell A4 contains LOOKUP (87,A1:F1)

Note that the numbers in A1:F1 are arranged in numeric order with the lowest number located in A1 and the highest in F1. If the numbers are not arranged that way LOOKUP will not work properly. When the Lookup function in cell A4 is executed SuperCalc will begin looking at the numbers in A1 through F1. It will "match" on 75 in D1 since it is the largest number that is "less than or equal to" the number in the Lookup parentheses. Then SuperCalc looks at the cell just below D1 (which is D2) and it displays the value in D2 (67) in cell A4.

**LN (#)**

Returns the natural log (log base e) of the number in the parentheses.

LN(3)=1.098612
LN(31)=3.433987

**LOG10 (#)**

Returns the log base 10 of the number in parentheses.

LOG10 (3)=.4771213
LOG10 (31)=1.491362

**MAX (LIST)**

This function looks at the list of cells specified in the parentheses. It finds the largest value and returns that value in the cell where the MAX function is located.

Here is an example:

A1-45 B1-48 C1-55 D1-75 E1-88 F1-97
A2-43 B2-03 C2-99 D2-67 E2-32 F2-03

In cell A4 type: MAX (A1:F1,C2,F2).

SuperCalc will look at cells A1 through F1 as well as cell C2 and cell F2. The largest number in this list of cells is 99 which is in cell C2. Cell A4 will thus contain 99.

### MIN (LIST)

This function looks at the list of cells specified in the parentheses. It finds the smallest value in the cells and returns that value in the cell where the MIN function is located.

Here is an example:

| | | | | | |
|---|---|---|---|---|---|
| A1-45 | B1-48 | C1-55 | D1-75 | E1-88 | F1-97 |
| A2-43 | B2-13 | C2-99 | D2-67 | E2-32 | F2-03 |

In cell A4 type: MIN (A1:F1,C2,F2).

SuperCalc will look at cells A1 through F1 as well as cell C2 and cell F2. The smallest number in this list of cells is 03, which is in cell F2. Cell A4 will thus contain 03.

### NPV (DISCOUNT, COL/ROW RANGE)

Net Present Value is the current value (or price) of cash flow which will become available in the future at specified time intervals. The discount in the parentheses takes into consideration the cost of the cash flow. NPV in SuperCalc assumes the column or row range specified contains numbers which indicate the cash flow that will occur at specified intervals. The discount specified is assumed to be for the interval reflected in the range, and all intervals are assumed to be equal. This is a complex function and Chapter 7 contains a complete example.

### PI

Using this function is the same as typing the value of PI with sixteen significant digits.

PI=3.141592653589793

### SIN (#), COS (#), TAN (#), ASIN (#), ACOS (#), ATAN (#)

These functions all return the value of the trigonometric functions of the numbers in parentheses. The value is given in radians. Sine, Cosine, Tangent, Arcsine, Arccosine, and Arctangent are available.

SIN(12)=−.536573
ATAN(PI)=1.262627

### SQRT (#)

Returns the square root of the number in the parentheses.

SQRT(4)=2
SQRT(81)=9

### SUM (LIST)

This function looks at the list of cells specified in the parentheses. It adds up the numbers found in those cells and returns that value in the cell where the Sum function is located. Here is an example:

| | | | | | |
|---|---|---|---|---|---|
| A1-45 | B1-48 | C1-55 | D1-75 | E1-88 | F1-97 |
| A2-43 | B2-03 | C2-99 | D2-67 | E2-32 | F2-03 |

In cell A4 type SUM (A1:F1,C2,F2).

SuperCalc will add up the numbers in A1 through F1 as well as cell C2 and cell F2. The sum or total is 510. Cell A4 will thus contain 510.

### CONDITIONAL EXPRESSIONS

Conditional expressions are a means of making decisions or comparisons. You may be familiar with conditional expressions in a different context as Boolean logic or Boolean algebra. All the conditional expressions let you make "Yes-No" or "True-False" decisions. There are four different types of conditional expressions (OR, AND, NOT, and IF) available in SuperCalc. There are standard formats for conditional expressions:

CONDITIONAL (Expression 1)
CONDITIONAL (Expression 1, Expression 2)
CONDITIONAL (Expression 1, Expression 2, Expression 3)

The conditional is one of the four noted above (OR, AND, NOT, IF). The expressions are calculations or comparisons that can be True (i.e., correct) or False (i.e., not correct). For example, A1=34 is an expression that may be true or false depending on the value of A1. The NOT conditional uses the one expression format, OR and AND use the two expression format, and IF uses either the two or three expression format.

The OR, AND, and NOT conditionals produce either a "1" or a "0" depending on whether expressions 1 and/or 2 are true or false. Here is the pattern:

| | |
|---|---|
| OR (TRUE, TRUE) | produces a 1 |
| OR (TRUE, FALSE) | produces a 1 |
| OR (FALSE, TRUE) | produces a 1 |
| OR (FALSE, FALSE) | produces a 0 |
| AND (TRUE, TRUE) | produces a 1 |
| AND (TRUE, FALSE) | produces a 0 |
| AND (FALSE, TRUE) | produces a 0 |
| AND (FALSE, FALSE) | produces a 0 |
| NOT (TRUE) | produces a 0 |
| NOT (FALSE) | produces a 1 |

An example would probably help:

A1-45 B1-48 C1-55 D1-75 E1-88 F1-97
A2-43 B2-03 C2-99 D2-67 E2-32 F2-03

In cell A4, type NOT(A1=45).

Cell A4 will display a 0 because the expression A1=45 is true and the rules for NOT specify that if the expression is true the value returned is a 0. Here are some more values for conditional expressions which are based on the cell values above.

IF (C1=55, D2=67) produces a 1
IF (C1=45, D2=64) produces a 0

OR (A2=43, F2=03) produces a 1
OR (B2=02, C2=99) produces a 1

**A More Complex Conditional Expression**

The IF conditional works in either the two or the three expression format. If expression 1 is correct, SuperCalc uses expression 2 for calculating the value in the cell where the IF conditional is placed. If expression 1 is not correct, SuperCalc uses expression 3 for calculating the value in the cell where the IF conditional is placed. Expression 3 is optional, and if not included, SuperCalc will use a value of 0 in the cell if expression 1 is not true. An example would probably help:

A1-45 B1-48 C1-55 D1-75 E1-88 F1-97
A2-43 B2-03 C2-99 D2-67 E2-32 F2-03

In cell A4, type IF (A1=45, B1*B2, B1/B2).

SuperCalc evaluates the expression A1=45. It is correct since cell A1 contains the value 45. Thus SuperCalc selects the second expression (B1*B2) and uses it to determine the value to be placed in cell A4. Cell A4 will thus contain 144 (48 times 3). If cell A4 had contained the conditional IF (A1=34, B1*B2, B1/B2) SuperCalc would use the third expression for calculating the value to be placed in C4 since A1 does not contain 34. Cell C4 would contain 16 (48 divided by 3).

In cell A4, type IF (A1=45, B1*B2)

Since this expression is true, SuperCalc uses the value of B1*B2 (144) as the value for the cell. If cell A1 had contained 35, the conditional would be false. Since expression 3 is omitted, SuperCalc would use a value of 0 in cell A4.

The three expression IF conditional is very flexible. You can even use other conditionals (AND, OR, NOT) in the first expression. Here is an example:

IF (NOT A1=B1, B1*B2, B1/B2)

Is the first expression correct? Correct is the same as true which is the same as returning a value of 1. NOT returns a value of 1 if the comparison (e.g., A1=B1) is not true. Thus NOT A1=B1 will be considered correct and the second expression (B1*B2 in this example) will be used instead of expression 3.

# Appendix

# Getting SuperCalc Up and Running

This appendix should be read *after* you have purchased SuperCalc and are ready to install it in your computer. Installing SuperCalc involves performing the preliminary steps required to create a diskette with both SuperCalc and CP/M on it that will run in your computer. SuperCalc runs on many different brands of computers, from ADDS to Zenith. Some of the computers use 5¼″ diskettes, others use 8″ diskettes. Even if two computers use the same size diskette, there may be differences in the method and format of storing information on the diskette. An 8″ diskette from a Cromemco, for example, will not necessarily run on a Xerox 820 computer with 8″ drives. To use SuperCalc, therefore, you must have a diskette with the program stored on it that is the correct size and uses the correct format. If you do not have the correct type of SuperCalc diskette, you must obtain one from your SuperCalc dealer before proceeding with the steps described in this appendix. We assume you have the following:

1. SuperCalc on a diskette that is the correct size and format for your computer.
2. CP/M on diskette for your computer. There are many versions of CP/M. SuperCalc will operate with CP/M version 2.2 or CP/M 86. (SuperCalc will also operate under other disk operating systems such as PC DOS for the IBM Personal Computer. See your dealer for information). Be sure you have a disk operating system that is compatible with SuperCalc before proceeding.
3. A CP/M compatible computer with at least 48K of RAM memory and disk drive. SuperCalc is distributed on diskette, and you must have at least one disk drive in order to be able to use SuperCalc.

### Note on Care of Diskettes

Although relatively sturdy, diskettes may be damaged if handled improperly. Do not place them on or near devices that might generate a magnetic field, avoid areas where excessive heat may build up (e.g., your glove compartment), and handle the diskettes only by their cover. Do not touch the thin platter inside the envelope since the oil on your fingers can ruin a diskette. Finally, always place the diskette in its paper carrier when not in use. Diskettes should, in fact, be stored in a protective box to keep them out of the dust, tobacco smoke, and pollution that occurs naturally (and not so naturally) in our environment.

In this appendix, we will provide a general outline of the steps needed to get SuperCalc "up and running" on your computer. Since the program runs on so many different computers, this section is, of necessity, somewhat general. When you buy the SuperCalc program, the package includes the correct diskette and a set of instructions for installing SuperCalc on your system. The material in this appendix will give you an idea of the steps required and their sequence. Directions provided in this appendix are appropriate for a CompuPro computer which has 64K of memory, two 8″ disk drives and CP/M 2.21. Other computers will vary somewhat in installation procedure, but will be similar. *Note:* Some dealers do the "install" for you and provide you with a version of SuperCalc that is ready to use with your system. If that is the case go directly to Step 5. All of the material in Steps 1-4 is explained in the users manual that comes with SuperCalc. This appendix will show you how to do the same things. This appendix gives you two opportunities to get the program up and running. If you still have problems, you may want to check *How to Get Started with CP/M* by Carl Townsend (dilithium Press).

### STEP 1. TURN ON COMPUTER AND LOAD CP/M

The CompuPro computer system can be turned on by pressing a switch on the front of the computer chassis. When the computer is on and the disk drive motors are spinning, a diskette with CP/M on it is placed in disk drive A. The computer will automatically load CP/M from the diskette into RAM in the computer. The video display will say something like this:

**CompuPro Disk1 System.**
**64K CP/M 2.21**

**A>**

The first line identifies your computer. The second line indicates that your version of CP/M is 2.21 and that it expects to be able to use 64K of memory (K=1024). Finally, the third line indicates CP/M considers drive A to be the primary or "system" drive and is ready to receive commands from you.

On some computers the disk drives are labeled with letters (e.g., A, B, C, or D), others use numbers (drive 1 is usually drive A under CP/M), and still others tell you which drive is "A" in the instruction manual, but not on the drives themselves. One way or another you will have to determine which of the drives in your system is drive A.

### STEP 2. MAKE A WORKING COPY OF CP/M

The procedure for making a copy of CP/M on a blank diskette varies considerably from system to system. The manuals that came with your copy of CP/M should help, as will the specific instructions for installing SuperCalc that came with the SuperCalc diskette. The CP/M diskette which was placed in drive A in Step 1 above should have CP/M on it, as well as programs called SUBMIT and PIP, and it should have at least 132K of space available for use. You can determine what is on the CP/M diskette by typing the command DIR and pressing the [RET] key (sometimes labeled the **ENTER** key) on your terminal or keyboard.

If everything is going according to plan, the computer will display a list of all the programs on the diskette in drive A on the screen. There will be several programs listed; two of them should be SUBMIT and PIP. If your copy of CP/M does not have these two programs on it, see your SuperCalc dealer for help.

Now, put a blank diskette in drive B (the other drive in a two drive system). You want to put a copy of CP/M (with PIP and SUBMIT) on this blank diskette. Later, SuperCalc will also be placed on this diskette. On our computer we must begin this process by "formatting" the new diskette. Some computer systems may call the process "initializing the diskette." Whatever the name, the process involves writing a sort of electronic map on the diskette. Later, when the computer wants to store data on the diskette, it will use the electronic map which was drawn during formatting as a guide to tell it where to place data. In our system, we can place the blank diskette in drive B, type the word Format and then press the [RET] key. The computer responds

**CompuPro Disk Sub-System FORMAT**
**Version 2.2B**
**Specify Drive (A:–D:) :**

The computer is asking us to tell it where the blank diskette is located (on drive A, B, C, or D). Since we put our blank diskette in drive B, we reply by pressing the B key. The computer responds

Disk is NOT formatted.
Select Disk format mode (0,1,2,3):
0=128  2=512
3=256  3=1024

The CompuPro computer can arrange or format the electronic map on the diskette in several different ways. It is asking us to tell it which of the four formats we want. We want the format specified by the number 3, so we press the 3 on the keyboard. Your computer may support fewer than four different formats. It may, in fact, support only one. If it can use only one format it will not ask you to specify a format mode. Instead, it will begin the process of formatting after you tell it which drive has the disk to be formatted. The CompuPro begins the formatting process by displaying this message:

**Confirm ready for format on disk drive B (y)**

This is your last chance to tell it you don't really want to format the diskette in B. This is a "failsafe" point since the formatting process erases everything that is stored on the diskette. If by accident, you told it to format a diskette that contains information you want to keep, this is your last chance to remove it from drive B and put a blank diskette in its place. If you do indeed have the correct diskette in B then press Y for Yes. If everything is going well, the computer will begin formatting the diskette. At this point, however, a common problem is likely to occur with novices and experienced computer operators alike. Instead of beginning to format the diskette, the computer may display this message:

**Disk does NOT have write ENABLED**
**Format error, do you want to continue (y)?**

Diskettes which contain valuable data can be "write protected" so that the disk drive will not write anything on the diskette even if directed to do so by the computer. On most 8″ diskettes there is a small notch at the end of the diskette which is opposite the label. This notch must be covered with a small stick-on label before the diskette can be "written to." Thus, 8″ diskettes with the notch are naturally write protected (that is, they don't come with the label placed over the notch). There is usually a supply of stick-on labels in each box of diskettes. If you have a system that uses the 5¼″ diskettes, the rules are just the opposite. There is a notch on the side of each diskette. If there is no label over that notch, the diskette can be formatted and used to store data. If the label is placed on it later, the diskette becomes "write protected" and, while the computer can read information already stored on it, additional data cannot be written onto the diskette.

Now, if you forgot to put the label on your 8″ diskette to be formatted (or to take it off a 5¼″ diskette), do it now. Then type Y for Yes in response to the question about continuing the formatting process. Our computer then asks

**Specify Drive (A:-D:) :**

Respond by pressing B again and we should be off and running. (It may also ask you several other questions again. Answer them the same way you did before.) During the formatting process our computer puts a row of numbers on the screen beginning with 0 and ending with 76. Then it places an "F" under each number as that part of the diskette is formatted. Our diskettes are divided into 77 tracks which are numbered from 0 to 76. After the computer finishes formatting all 77 tracks, it goes back and verifies each track. Verification involves checking to see if the electronic map of each track has been correctly drawn. As each track is verified the computer places a "V" under the track number.

When formatting is complete, the computer will ask you what you want to do next. Ours lets us choose between formatting another diskette and going back to CP/M (exit back to system). We want to get back to CP/M, so we press N which is the code letter beside "exit back to system."

### Now: Put a Copy of CP/M on Your Formatted Diskette

At this point there is a properly formatted diskette in drive B and a CP/M diskette in drive A. Our version of CP/M has a program called COPY which can be used to create a duplicate of any diskette in drive A on the diskette in drive B. To begin the process, type

COPY (and then press the [RET] key)

The computer replies

**CompPro COPY Utility Version 2.4.**
**Do you want to copy:**
**SYSTEM tracks only? (type S)**
**DATA tracks only? (type D)**
**ALL of the disk? (type A)**
**Exit back to System? (type X)**

The computer can select all or only part of the information on the diskette in A to be copied over to B. You may well want to use that capability later. For the moment tell the computer you want ALL of the diskette copied by pressing A on the keyboard. The computer then asks

**Source drive? (A,B,C, or D)**

Press the A key since that is where the original or *source* diskette is located. The source diskette is the diskette which contains the information or data you want to copy. The computer will now ask

**Destination drive (A,B,C,orD)**

Press the B key because the diskette where the copy will be placed is in drive B. The computer will reply with

**Put source disk on A**
**Put destination disk on B**
**Then type** [RET]

You already have your diskettes in the correct drives, so the next step is to press the [RET] key (don't type R-E-T-U-R-N). When the [RET] key is pressed, the computer will begin the copying process. It takes the information on each sector of the diskette in drive A, reads it into the memory of the computer, and then duplicates that information on the same sector on the diskette in drive A. It does not "remove" the information on diskette A, it "copies" the information to diskette B. That means you will have two identical diskettes when the process is completed.

As the computer does its work, it may list the number of the sector being copied on the screen, and it will tell you when the copy process is complete:

**COPY Complete.**
**Do you want to COPY again? (Y/N)**

You don't want to make another copy, so press the **N** key. The computer responds with

**Remount system disk on A: and type RETURN**

Take the copy you made from drive B and put it in drive A. Take the original CP/M diskette in drive A and put it in a safe place. Now press the [RET] key. The computer will respond

**A>**

It is telling you that CP/M is now ready to accept further instructions and that the primary or *system* drive is currently drive A.

## STEP 3. PUT A COPY OF SUPERCALC ON YOUR CP/M DISKETTE

Now we get down to the nitty gritty. It is time to put SuperCalc on your diskette and start using it! First, put the copy of CP/M you made in Step 2 in drive A. (Take the original or source diskette for CP/M that was in drive A and put it in a safe place.) Now, put the "distribution" diskette with SuperCalc on it in drive B. The distribution diskette is the one that came with the SuperCalc package from the dealer. That diskette contains a special "install" program that copies all the SuperCalc programs on it to the disk in drive A, which already contains CP/M. Once this step is completed, you will have a working copy of SuperCalc on a disk that contains the CP/M operating system. It will be ready to work for you. With the SuperCalc disk in drive B and the CP/M diskette in drive A, type the following:

[CTL] **C**

That is, find the key labeled **CONTROL** or **CTRL** on your keyboard. Press and hold it down. While the [CTL] key is held down, press the C key as well. The [CTL] C instruction tells the computer to log in the current disks (they may already be logged in, but go ahead and type [CTL] C anyway just to be sure). When the computer responds with another A>, type the following:

**SUBMIT B:INSTALL** (and press the [RET] key)

When the computer gets the instructions above, it will look for a program called INSTALL on drive B, load it into memory, and begin following the instructions. As those instructions are executed the computer will take the SuperCalc programs on diskette B and copy them over to diskette A. As it does this, the screen will give you a running description of what is happening. If it occasionally says NO FILE, don't worry; it is supposed to do that. When it is finished you will have a working SuperCalc program on the diskette in drive A. Take the distribution diskette (in drive B) and store it in a safe place. You will not use the distribution diskette again, *unless* you damage or destroy all your copies of SuperCalc and have to go through this INSTALL process again (heaven forbid). Also, if you wish to order a new version of SuperCalc in the future, you may be asked to send the distribution diskette to the dealer for updating.

Now take the diskette out of drive A and label it using the stick-on labels that came in the box with the diskettes. We usually write "SC CP/M" on ours with a felt tip pen. Don't use a pencil or a ball point pen since the pressure of the tip might damage the diskette's magnetic surface. Even better, write the title on the label before applying it to the diskette.

## STEP 4. MAKE ANY CHANGES REQUIRED BY YOUR SYSTEM

In this step you will make any changes required to make your copy of SuperCalc run on your computer. You will need to tell SuperCalc which computer you are using. Some computers require the use of a separate *terminal* which contains the video display and keyboard. You could, for example, purchase a NorthStar Horizon computer and use it with a Lear Seigler ADM-3A terminal, a DEC VT-52 terminal, a Televidio 910, or any of over 50 other terminals. That means just having SuperCalc for the NorthStar is not enough. You must tell SuperCalc which brand and model of terminal you are using as well as the brand and model of computer. (The saving grace of all this is that you only have to do it once.) Thus, you must complete one more step. Put the SuperCalc CP/M diskette in drive A, type [CTL] C to be sure the disks are logged in, and then type the following:

INSTALL (and press the RET key)

The computer will reply with

**SUPERCALC Install Program**
**Version : 1.25**

This program will install your SuperCalc file for the terminal that you wish to use.

**Do you wish to proceed (n/y)?**

Type Y in response to the question above. SuperCalc will reply with

**Enter name of SuperCalc (tm) file as:**
**"d:filename" where "d" is the drive.**
**Enter ? for more help.**
**Enter name:**

Since you have SuperCalc in the A drive and it is named SC.COM (why is it named that? Because the programmer named it SC and CP/M added .COM to it as an "extension"), you should type the following:

A:SC.COM (and press RET)

When the RET key is pressed, SuperCalc will read some information in the SuperCalc program into memory and then put a list of the terminals supported by SuperCalc on the video display. At the bottom of the screen the following line appears:

**Enter A–O, Y, Z, or ?**

SuperCalc is asking you to select a letter to indicate your wishes. At the top of the screen is the name of the terminal currently supported. Below that is a list of several other brands of terminals. Is the one you will be using listed there? If it is, type in the letter beside it and press the RET key. If, for example, you will be using a Hazeltine terminal, press E and RET.

What if your terminal isn't listed? The material that came with your copy of SuperCalc includes a list of many other terminals. The list indicates, for example, that the ABM80 terminal works like the DEC VT-52 terminal. If you have an ABM80, tell SuperCalc you have a DEC (option D on the screen) and SuperCalc will be happy.

If your terminal is not listed on either the screen or the sheet included in the material that comes with SuperCalc, you should stop here and see your SuperCalc dealer for assistance. Most dealers have the facilities to set up SuperCalc to run on your terminal.

Let's assume, however, that the brand of your terminal is found on the screen or in the INSTALL material. If you haven't already done so, press the letter indicating the terminal (or equivalent). If there are several different models of the brand of terminal you will be using, SuperCalc will now list the different models on the screen and ask you to press a key indicating the model you will be using. Do that now. Then SuperCalc will give you some more options:

**This is what you may now do:**
**A. Save SuperCalc on disk.**
**B. Return to first menu.**
**C. Quit Install Program.**
**Enter A,B,or C or ?:**

Select the A option (press the A key). Then SuperCalc will tell you which terminal was selected and give you one more chance to correct any errors. If everything is fine, press Y. SuperCalc will modify the program to run correctly with your terminal and display the message:

**You may now use your SUPERCALC(tm) program**

### STEP 5. ONE MORE THING

If the SuperCalc program is still in drive A, you could begin using it right now. It is only necessary to type:

SC (and press the RET key)

and you are off and running! After all the work to get to this point, it is certainly a temptation to do just that. Persevere just a few more moments. It is good practice to *backup* your diskettes so that damage to one will not mean the only copy of a program or important data is lost. While this section was being written (in West Texas) there was a severe thunderstorm and several tornado warnings. During a particularly hard rain (accompanied by large hail that covered the ground), the power to our building was knocked out several times by nearby lightning. Each time power was lost, the material in the computer's memory was lost. In addition, lightning also caused a "spike" to come into the computer on the power line and damage one of the diskettes we were using. Fortunately, we had a backup of the diskette. The material in memory was lost, however, and had to be entered again. A *backup diskette* is simply a duplicate of a diskette you are using. Very important data or programs should probably be backed up several times.

Before using the SuperCalc diskette you just created for actual work, back it up (several times). Then if something happens (the dog takes a diskette out in the yard and buries it, the kids spill hot chocolate on it, or a boozy friend looks at it too closely and irrigates it with Bailey's Irish Cream) you will have a replacement. You can make a backup of your diskette by following the directions given in Step 2.

It is time to start learning how to use SuperCalc now. After your backups are made, proceed to the Tutorial Section and Happy Computing!

# Index

# ABOUT THE AUTHORS

Deborrah Smithy-Willis, Jerry Willis and Merl Miller are all accomplished computerists and well-known authors.

Deborrah Smithy-Willis has a doctorate in Education Psychology. She does workshops and seminars on computer literacy and is a consultant to businesses and schools on the subject of microcomputers. She is the co-author of *Peanut Butter and Jelly Guide to Computers.*

Jerry Willis is the author of such books as *Nailing Jelly to a Tree, Peanut Butter and Jelly Guide to Computers* and *Computers for Everybody*, first and second editions – and all were chosen by the Library Journal as outstanding computer publications. Jerry holds a masters degree in education and a doctorate in clinical psychology. He is currently a professor in Educational Psychology at Texas Tech.

Merl Miller is an industrial engineer who got involved in computers and electronics as a hobby. He is a graduate of the University of Wyoming and has been publishing books for 14 years. Merl has written such books as *Computers for Everybody*, first and second editions, *How to Make Money With Your Microcomputer*, and *From the Counter to the Bottom Line.* Merl is currently the Chairman of the Board for dilithium Press.